Complications in Orthopaedics
Pediatric Upper Extremity Fractures

Edited by
Charles T. Price, MD
Surgeon in Chief
Pediatric Orthopaedics
Nemours Children's Clinic
Orlando, Florida

Series Editor
Jeffrey O. Anglen, MD
Boone Orthopaedic Associates
Columbia, Missouri

Published by the
American Academy of Orthopaedic Surgeons
6300 North River Road
Rosemont, IL 60018

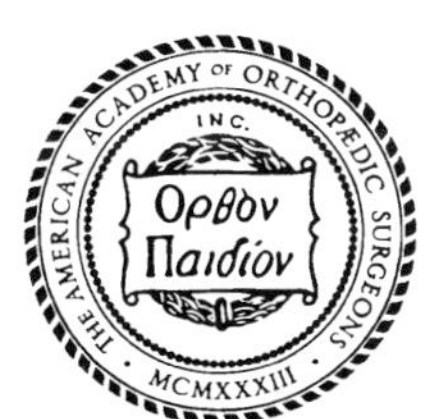

American Academy of Orthopaedic Surgeons

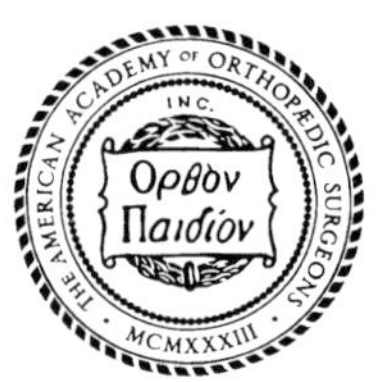

American Academy of Orthopaedic Surgeons Board of Directors, 2004

American Academy of Orthopaedic Surgeons
6300 North River Road
Rosemont, IL 60018
1-800-626-6726

The material presented in *Pediatric Upper Extremity Fractures* has been made available by the American Academy of Orthopaedic Surgeons for educational purposes only. This material is not intended to present the only, or necessarily best, methods or procedures for the medical situations discussed, but rather is intended to represent an approach, view, statement, or opinion of the author(s) or producer(s), which may be helpful to others who face similar situations.

Some drugs or medical devices demonstrated in Academy courses or described in Academy print or electronic publications have not been cleared by the Food and Drug Administration (FDA) or have been cleared for specific uses only. The FDA has stated that it is the responsibility of the physician to determine the FDA clearance status of each drug or device he or she wishes to use in clinical practice.

PMMA bone cement is considered a device for FDA purposes. In October 1999, the FDA reclassified PMMA bone cement as a Class II device for its intended use "in arthroplastic procedures of the hip, knee, and other joints for the fixation of polymer or metallic prosthetic implants to living bone." The use of a device for other than its FDA-cleared indication is an off-label use. Physicians may use a device off-label if they believe, in their best medical judgment, that its use is appropriate for a particular patient (eg, tumors).

Furthermore, any statements about commercial products are solely the opinion(s) of the author(s) and do not represent an Academy endorsement or evaluation of these products. These statements may not be used in advertising or for any commercial purpose.

First Edition

ISBN 0-89203-331-2

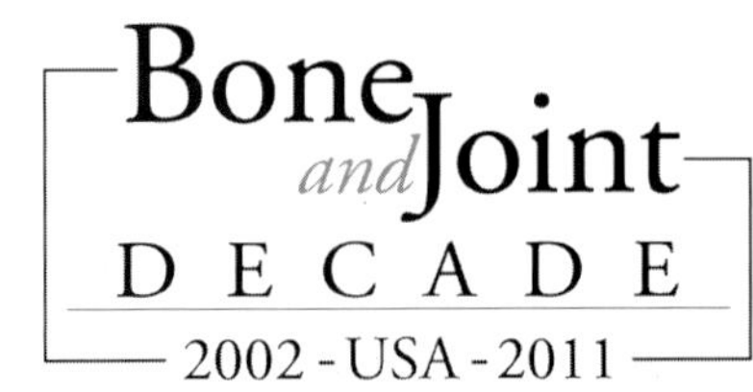

Contributors

John M. Flynn, MD
Associate Professor of Orthopaedic Surgery
Department of Orthopaedic Surgery
The Children's Hospital of Philadelphia
Philadelphia, Pennsylvania

Kenneth J. Noonan, MD
Associate Professor
Department of Orthopaedics
Department of Pediatrics
University of Wisconsin
Madison, Wisconsin

Charles T. Price, MD
Surgeon in Chief
Nemours Children's Clinic
Orlando, Florida

Peter M. Waters, MD
Director, Hand and Upper Extremity Surgery
Children's Hospital
Department of Orthopaedic Surgery
Boston, Massachusetts

Contents

Preface

Approximately 2% of children sustain a fracture each year. Boys have a 40% risk and girls a 25% risk of sustaining a fracture of some type from birth to age 16 years.[1] Because upper extremity fractures account for 70% to 75% of all limb fractures in children,[1,2] it is especially important for orthopedic surgeons to understand their management and the complications that can result from these fractures.

Some complications are preventable; most can be corrected with proper secondary management. Unfortunately, litigation is common for fracture complications in children. A review of Physicians Insurers Association of America claims data from 1985 to 2000 for orthopaedic conditions affecting patients younger than age 18 years indicates that 77% of all orthopaedic litigation in this age group stems from fracture care. Most of these claims are resolved in favor of the physician; however, the stated reasons for most of these complaints are improper treatment, misdiagnosis, and missed complications.

The elbow, proximal forearm, and hand are at high risk for fracture complications. Accurate diagnosis may be difficult when using plain radiographs for fractures in these regions. When malunion occurs, these regions of slow growth have little potential for remodeling. Nonunion is also a potential complication for intra-articular fractures around the elbow, even though nonunions are uncommon in children. Anatomic reduction and surgical stabilization are frequently required for fractures in these regions of high risk. Growth disturbances from physeal arrest can occur around the elbow or hand but rarely lead to serious deformity. In contrast, growth arrest of the distal radius or ulna is likely to require treatment.

Misdiagnosis may occur with fractures around the elbow and hand for a variety of reasons. Misdiagnosis of radial head dislocation in Monteggia injury is often the result of a perceptual error on the part of the physician. Much attention in radiology literature has been directed to perceptual errors. One common cause, identified as "satisfaction of search,"[3] occurs when the detection of one abnormality reduces the chance of identifying additional abnormalities. This effect may occur in Monteggia lesions when the fracture is identified as the cause of deformity and pain, but the physician overlooks the radial head dislocation and treats only the fracture.

Another cause of misdiagnosis of elbow fractures in children is the predominantly cartilaginous composition of the distal humerus. Multiple ossification centers that appear at different ages may add to the diagnostic dilemma. Radiographs of injured pediatric elbows may demonstrate small fragments of bone that appear to be minor avulsion injuries when the true fracture involves a much larger segment of cartilage. Medial condyle fracture is easily misdiagnosed as a medial epicondylar avulsion prior to ossification of the trochlea. The medial epicondyle ossifies at an average age of 7 years, whereas the ossification center of the trochlea does not appear until an average age of 9 years. During this period of time in particular, the appearance of a medial epicondyle fracture should arouse suspicion of a medial condyle fracture.

Any swelling or restriction of motion following an elbow injury to a child should prompt a thorough search for serious injury. Plain radiographs may be insufficient for accurate diagnosis; special imaging techniques that define cartilage provide the greatest amount of information. The most useful imaging techniques are MRI, ultrasonography, and arthrography. Ultrasonography is primarily applicable for infants and very young children.[4] Comparison radiographs may help identify variations of normal but add little to the diagnostic accuracy.[5] Magnification and

CT techniques also add little to conventional radiography for pediatric elbow fractures.[6,7]

Complications may also develop as a result of inadequate posttreatment radiographs or inadequate follow-up. An entrapped intra-articular medial epicondyle can occur following reduction of elbow dislocation. This may be very difficult to identify due to cast or splint materials or to elbow position. When in doubt, radiographs without immobilization should be obtained. The risk of losing reduction is generally less than the risk of inadequate treatment of a continuing problem. Radiographs of fractures should be orthogonal to the fractured bone. For example, in the case of a supracondylar fracture it would be more accurate to request AP and lateral radiographs of the distal humerus than to request AP and lateral radiographs of the elbow because elbow views may produce inadequate radiographs of a child immobilized in a cast.

Common sources of inadequate follow-up include patient noncompliance, miscommunication with office staff responsible for return appointments, and failure to recommend return in a timely manner. When in doubt, it is better to err on the side of frequent follow-up. Follow-up of multitrauma patients should include review of radiographs and reexamination of the patient a few days following the initial trauma to detect occult injuries that were not apparent at the time of presentation.

Cast problems are another source of general complications in pediatric upper extremity fractures. Constrictive casts may help maintain alignment but can contribute to vascular compromise in the presence of postreduction edema. Bivalved casts are recommended postoperatively to allow for swelling. Changing casts in a timely manner as swelling subsides will allow maintenance of alignment. Supervision of assistants may be necessary for cast removal when the cast has become wet, swelling is still present, or padding has been removed by small children.

Neurovascular complications are the most serious complications that occur with any frequency and have been identified as a particular area of risk. A pearl that might help reduce the incidence of these complications comes from the AAOS Committee on Professional Liability:[8] "There is no such thing as a hypochondriac in a cast; listen to complaints."

I would like to acknowledge the assistance of the authors who have contributed their expertise to this monograph. I also would like to thank the Academy Publications Department, especially Lynne Shindoll, Managing Editor, and Joan Abern, Senior Editor, for their assistance in bringing this project to fruition.

Charles T. Price, MD
Editor

References

1. Tiderius CJ, Landin L, Henrik D: Decreasing incidence of fractures in children. *Acta Orthop Scand* 1999;70:622-626.
2. Cheng JCY, Shen WY: Limb fracture patterns in different pediatric age groups: A study of 3,350 children. *J Orthop Trauma* 1993;7:15-22.
3. Ashman CJ, Yu JS, Wolfman D: Satisfaction of search in osteoradiology. *AJR Am J Roentgenol* 2000;175:541-544.
4. Davidson RS, Markowitz RI, Dormans J, Drummond DS: Ultrasonographic evaluation of the elbow in infants and young children after suspected trauma. *J Bone Joint Surg Am* 1994;76:1804-1813.
5. Kissoon N, Galpin R, Gayle M, Chacon D, Brown T: Evaluation of the role of comparison radiographs in the diagnosis of traumatic elbow injuries. *J Ped. Orthop* 1995;15:449-453.
6. Blickman JG, Dunlop RW, Sanzone CF, Franklin PD: Is CT useful in the traumatized pediatric elbow? *Pediatr Radiol* 1990;20:184-185.
7. Holland P, Davies AM, Morris E, Fowler J, Wellings R, Tyrrell PNM: Real-time digital contrast enhancement and magnification in the assessment of acute elbow injuries. *Br J Radiol* 1991;64:591-595.
8. AAOS Committee on Professional Liability: *Managing Orthopaedic Malpractice*, ed 2. Rosemont, IL, American Academy of Orthopaedic Surgeons, 2000.

Chapter 1

Phalangeal Fracture Malunion

Peter M. Waters, MD

Case Presentation

History

A 4-year-old girl who caught her middle finger in a door had swelling, ecchymosis, limited active range of motion, and guarding in the affected finger on examination in the emergency department. Initial radiographs showed a minor phalangeal fracture (Figure 1) for which she was placed in a single digit splint. Her parents were told to remove the splint after 5 to 7 days and to expect her fracture to heal without difficulties. They were also advised to seek hand consultation only if there was persistent swelling. Fifteen days after the injury, the patient was examined in the hand clinic with persistent pain and swelling.

Current Problem and Treatment

Examination in the hand clinic revealed fusiform swelling of the affected finger, active motion in the proximal interphalangeal (PIP) joint of 45°, and passive motion of 60°. The finger was not tender to compression and percussion manipulation at the fracture site, and there was a healed palpable callus. Radiographs obtained at this time revealed a displaced proximal phalangeal neck fracture in extension that showed a moderate degree of healing (Figure 2). The proximal metaphyseal fracture fragment was blocking the subchondral fossa. Because there was persistent lucency at the fracture site, immediate surgical intervention was indicated.

With the patient under general anesthesia and the finger under fluoroscopic imaging, closed reduction was attempted but not possible because the fracture fragment was not mobile. There was a firm block to flexion at 55° where the volar aspect of the middle phalanx abutted the proximal phalangeal metaphyseal fragment. Concerns about osteonecrosis with open reduction led to first attempt a percutaneous osteoclasis. A smooth 0.45-in cerclage wire was inserted obliquely, under fluoroscopic guidance, into the fracture site to avoid the central extensor mechanism (Figure 3). Manipulative reduction was then attempted by levering the fracture fragment into flexion. After reduction, full passive flexion of the interphalangeal (IP) joint to 105° was possible. Percutaneous pinning of the fracture into the corrected position followed. Postoperatively, the finger was immobilized 4 weeks followed by in-office pin removal. Full active and passive motion was restored by 6 weeks after surgery.

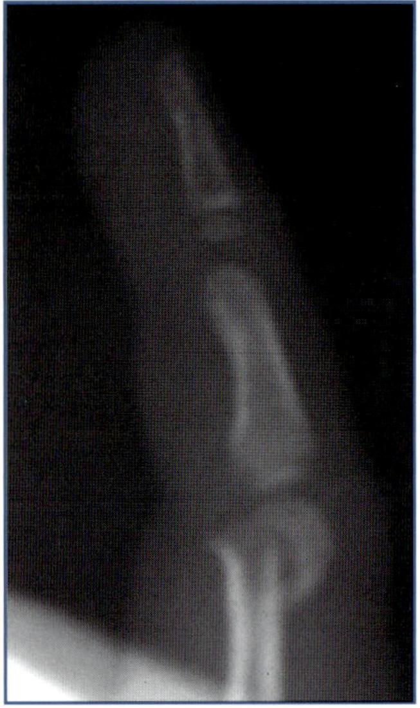

Figure 1 Example case: Acute phalangeal neck fracture with extension deformity. Too often the severity of this fracture is underestimated in the acute setting.

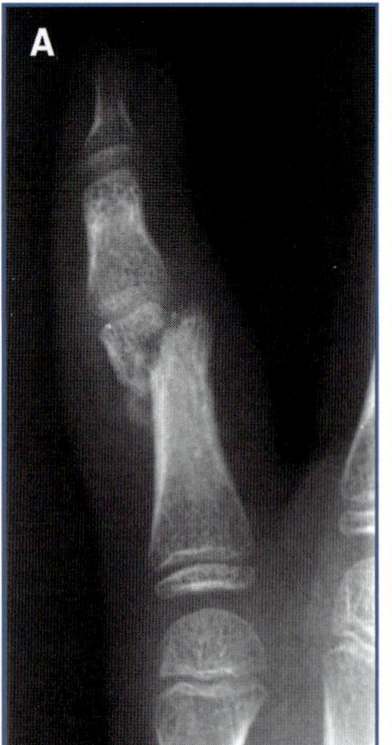

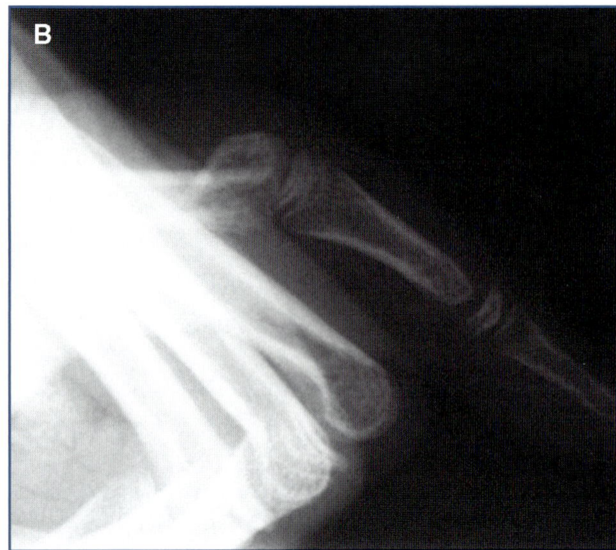

Figure 2 Example case: Preoperative AP **(A)** and lateral **(B)** radiographs of late presenting phalangeal neck fracture with an incipient malunion and loss of IP joint flexion.

Discussion

Recognizing the Problem and Situations at High Risk

Approximately 75% to 80% of pediatric hand fractures are uncomplicated and will have an excellent result in terms of alignment and restoration of motion, function, and strength.[1-5] Treatment of the simple, nondisplaced fracture should include protective immobilization until healing, followed by return to unrestricted activities. It is imperative, however, to immediately recognize potentially hazardous fractures. These include (1) intercondylar phalangeal fractures; (2) phalangeal and metacarpal shaft fractures with malrotation; (3) phalangeal neck fractures; (4) displaced physeal fractures (Salter-Harris type III fractures of the thumb or finger metacarpophalangeal joint, Seymour fractures of the distal phalanx, or Salter-Harris type II proximal phalanx fractures); and (5) intra-articular osteochondral fractures.[1-6] All of these fractures require reduction and stabilization to prevent a suboptimal result.

Management of Malunion

Malunion is the most common serious complication among pediatric hand fractures. Too often malunion results from failure to recognize the problematic fracture in the acute care setting. With fracture malunion, the delay in referral or intervention leads to loss of motion and function. Most of these problematic fractures will not remodel.

With a phalangeal neck fracture, the distal fragment displaces into extension.[1,2,7,8] The collateral ligaments of the IP joint maintain stability and vascularity to the fragment.[9] The proximal metaphyseal fragment occludes the volar subchondral fossa and blocks interphalangeal flexion[7,8,10,11] (Figure 4). Closed reduction is effected with distraction and then flexion of the displaced condylar fragment. Any element of malrotation or malangulation should be corrected with the distraction maneuver, restoring full passive interphalangeal flexion. If the problem is recognized early, closed reduction and percutaneous pin stabilization can lead to anatomic healing and full restoration of function. Small, smooth pins are placed obliquely from the radial and ulnar condyles in an oblique, distal to proximal, fashion across the fracture site. The pins are removed at 3 to 4 weeks with radiographic evidence of healing.

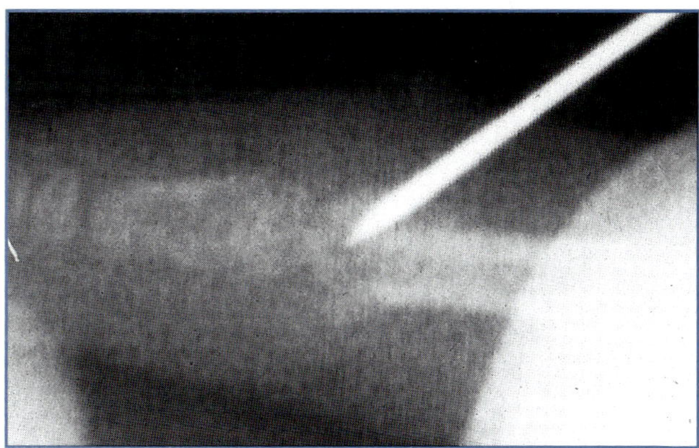

Figure 3 Example case: Lateral intraoperative fluoroscopic image of percutaneous reduction of the incipient malunion.

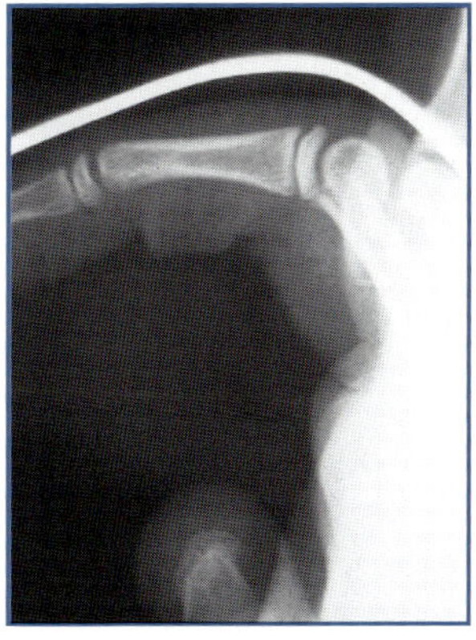

Figure 4 Phalangeal neck fracture with persistent malalignment after attempted closed reduction. This fracture requires anatomic reduction and pinning. (Reproduced with permission from Waters PM: The upper limb, in Morrissy RT, Weinstein SK (eds): *Lovell and Winter's Pediatric Orthopedics*, ed 5. Philadelphia, PA, Lippincott-Williams & Wilkins, 2001, vol 2, pp 841-903.)

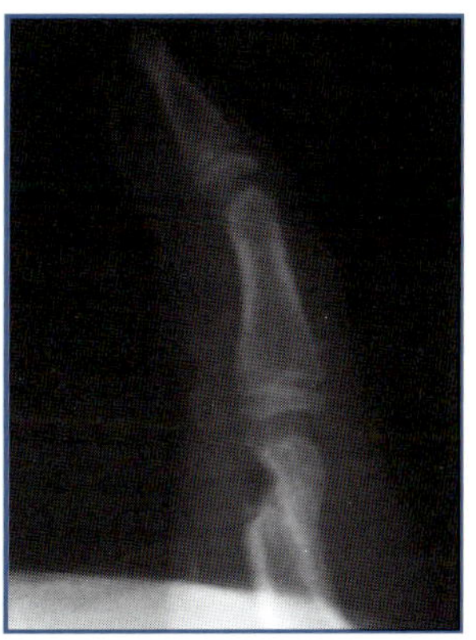

Figure 5 Subchondral fossa reconstruction of a proximal phalangeal neck malunion with a preoperative block to flexion at 50° and postoperative proximal interphalangeal flexion to 95°.

Permanent restriction of interphalangeal motion is a concern with any periarticular fracture, especially at the PIP joint. Therefore, aggressive home or supervised therapy is indicated after these fractures, even in the setting of anatomic healing.

Occasionally these fractures cannot be reduced in the semiacute setting. In these cases, open reduction through a midaxial incision is indicated. The dorsal extensor mechanism is preserved and elevated, and the volar neurovascular bundle is protected. Care also must be taken to preserve the collateral ligament to prevent osteonecrosis of the distal fracture fragment. Reduction of the fracture fragment occurs with digital flexion at the involved IP joint. The subchondral fossa is restored in the operating room, resulting in full passive interphalangeal flexion. Pin stabilization is the same as with closed reduction.

More often than desired, children with phalangeal malunion do not present until advanced bony healing has occurred, after which time closed reduction and percutaneous pinning is no longer a viable option. If radiolucency remains at the fracture line, percutaneous pin osteoclasis can be performed.[12] A smooth pin is placed from dorsal obliquely into the fracture site under fluoroscopic control, avoiding the central extensor mechanism. The pin is used to lever the fracture volarly, restoring the subchondral fossa, in a fashion similar to that used in adult distal radius fractures or pediatric radial neck fractures.[13,14]

If the fracture is completely healed, treatment options include osteotomy, subchondral fossa reconstruction,[15] and remodeling.[16-18] The principal concern with early osteotomy is osteonecrosis. Care must be taken to preserve the precarious blood supply to the distal fragment through the collateral ligaments.[9] Reconstruction of the subchondral fossa has been advocated 6 months or more after malunion to improve flexion of the IP joint. Note that reconstruction improves but does not normalize flexion of the IP joint. By a volar approach, the subchondral region is débrided of metaphyseal bone until passive flexion of more than 90° is achieved (Figure 5). Early postoperative therapy is necessary to maintain the corrected motion.

Remodeling of phalangeal neck fractures rarely has been described (Figure 6). The phalangeal physis is proximal, and the malunion is distal. Therefore, most authors state that remodeling is not feasible.[7,8] However, profound remodeling has been reported in young

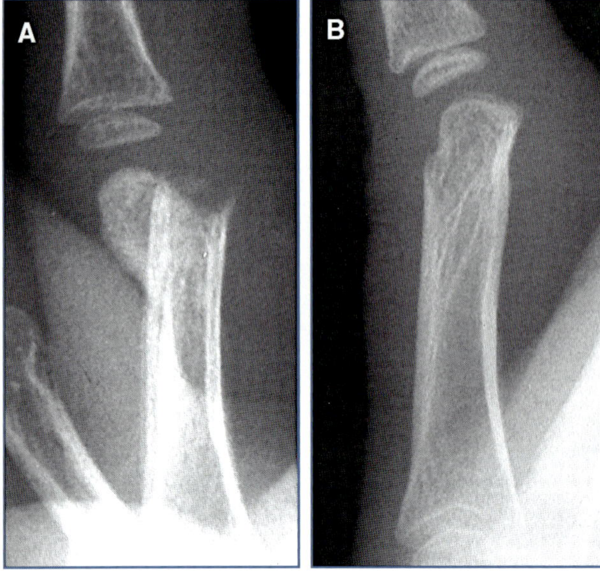

Figure 6 Remodeling of a phalangeal neck fracture malunion over a 2-year period. Initial radiograph **(A)** showing loss of the subchondral fossa and proximal interphalangeal flexion. **B,** Restoration of the fossa 2 years later with full motion.

children more than 1 to 2 years after the fracture occurs. If the joint surface is congruent, there is no malrotation, there are many years of growth remaining, and the family and patient can tolerate a prolonged time for slow improvement, then remodeling may be appropriate. Clearly, the best treatment for a phalangeal neck malunion is prevention. Early diagnosis with reduction and stabilization is the treatment of choice.

Preventing Malunion

Radiographic recognition of problematic fractures is critical to preventing malunion. True AP and lateral radiographs are necessary to identify displaced fractures. Clinical examination for malrotation with passive tenodesis (Figure 7) and active motion in the cooperative child is important, regardless of the radiographic appearance. Significant clinical malrotation can occur when radiographs appear benign. In the acute or semiacute setting, all hand fractures should be assessed for malrotation to prevent malunion. Appropriate referral or surgical intervention should occur

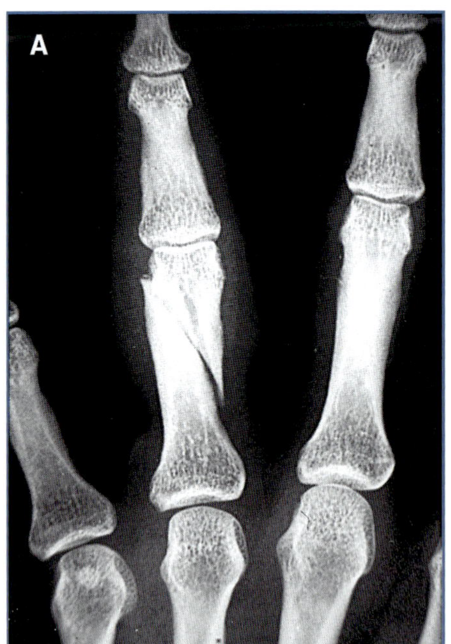

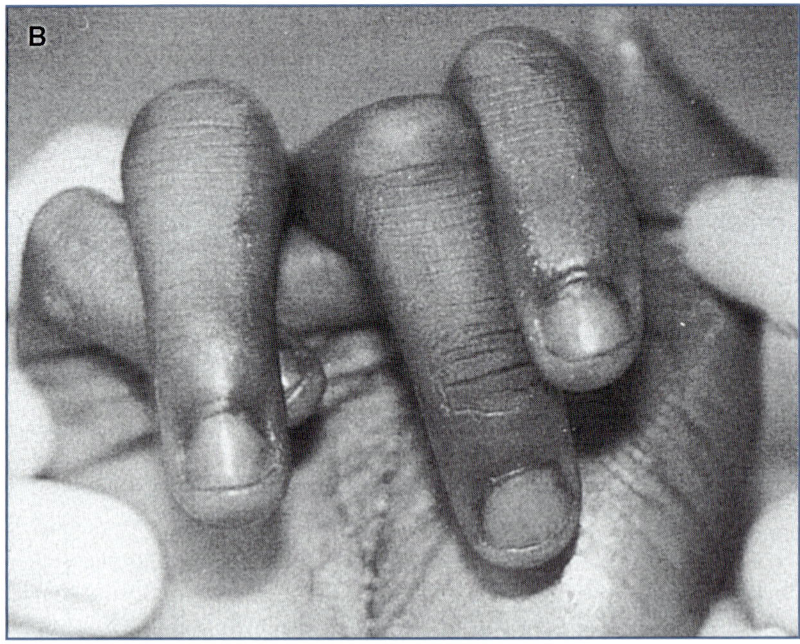

Figure 7 A, Displaced proximal phalanx fracture with malrotation. **B,** Tenodesis testing revealing malrotation. By passively extending and flexing the wrist, the digits will passively flex and extend, respectively. Malalignment is evident. (Reproduced with permission from Waters PM: The upper limb, in Morrissy RT, Weinstein SK (eds): *Lovell and Winter's Pediatric Orthopedics*, ed 5. Philadelphia, PA, Lippincott-Williams & Wilkins, 2001, vol 2, pp 841-903.)

within the first 3 to 7 days for these problematic fractures before advanced bony healing occurs.

CASE MANAGEMENT AND OUTCOME SUMMARY

In this case, percutaneous reduction of the partially healed fracture was performed (Figure 3) followed by pin stabilization. The fracture was immobilized in a cast for 4 weeks until complete healing. The pin was removed and postoperative therapy begun. Fortunately, motion and function were completely restored although this patient was at risk for loss of IP joint flexion.

REFERENCES

1. Graham TJ, Hastings H: Management of fractured fingers in the child, in Gupta A, Kay SPJ, Schecker LR (eds): *The Growing Hand.* London, England, Harcourt, 2000, pp 591-607.
2. Graham TJ, Waters PM: Fractures and dislocations of the hand and carpus in children, in Beaty JH, Kasser JR (eds): *Rockwood and Wilkins' Fractures in Children*, ed 5. Philadelphia, PA, Lippincott-Williams & Wilkins, 2001, pp 269-379.
3. Armstrong PF, Joughin VE, Clarke HM: Pediatric fractures of the forearm, wrist, and hand, in Green NE, Swiontkowski MF (eds): *Skeletal Trauma in Children,* ed 2. Philadelphia, PA, Saunders, 1998, pp 161-257.
4. Green DP: Hand injuries in children. *Pediatr Clin North Am* 1977;24:903-918.
5. Fischer MD, McElfresh EC: Physeal and periphyseal injuries of the hand: Patterns of injury and results of treatment. *Hand Clin* 1994;10:287-301.
6. Hastings H, Simmons BP: Hand fractures in children: A statistical analysis. *Clin Orthop* 1984;188:120-130.
7. Barton NJ: Fractures of the phalanges of the hand in children. *Hand* 1979;11:134-143.
8. Barton NJ: Fractures of the shafts of the phalanges of the hand. *Hand* 1979;11:119-133.
9. Yousif NJ, Cunningham MW, Sanger JR, Gingrass RP, Matloub HS: The vascular supply to the proximal interphalangeal joint. *J Hand Surg [Am]* 1985;10:852-861.
10. Al-Qattan MM: Phalangeal neck fractures in children: Classification and outcome in 66 cases. *J Hand Surg [Br]* 2001;26:112-121.
11. Leonard MH, Dubravcik P: Management of fractured fingers in the child. *Clin Orthop* 1970;73:160-168.
12. Waters PM: The upper limb, in Morrissy RT, Weinstein SK (eds) *Lovell and Winter's Pediatric Orthopaedics.* Philadelphia, PA, Lippincott Williams & Wilkins, 2001, vol 2, pp 887-888.
13. Bernstein SM, McKeever P, Bernstein L: Percutaneous reduction of displaced radial neck fractures in children. *J Pediatr Orthop* 1993;13:85-88.
14. Trumbe TE, Wagner W, Hanel DP, Vedder NB, Gilbert M: Intrafocal (Kapandji) pinning of distal radius fractures with and without external fixation. *J Hand Surg [Am]* 1998;23:381-394.
15. Simmons BP, Peters TT: Subcondylar fossa reconstruction for malunion of fractures of the proximal phalanx in children. *J Hand Surg [Am]* 1987;12:1079-1082.
16. Hennirkus WL, Cohen MR: Complete remodeling of displaced fractures of the neck of the phalanx. *J Bone Joint Surg Br* 2003;85:273-274.
17. Mintzer CM, Waters PM, Brown DJ: Remodelling of a displaced phalangeal neck fracture. *J Hand Surg [Br]* 1994;19:594-596.
18. Ogden JA, Ganey TM, Ogden DA: The biological aspects of children's fractures, in Rockwood CA, Wilkins KE, Beaty JH (eds): *Fractures in Children*, ed 4. Philadelphia, PA, Lippincott-Raven, 1996, pp 19-52.

Chapter 2

Ulnar Growth Arrest After Distal Radius and Ulna Fracture

Kenneth J. Noonan, MD

Case Presentation

History

A right-handed 10-year-old boy sustained a metaphyseal fracture of the right distal radius and a fracture of the ulnar metaphysis with extension into the ulnar growth plate as a result of a fall (Figure 1). After attempted closed reduction, the radius could not be completely reduced and remained bayonet opposed with 100% displacement. The reduction was accepted because no angulation was present, and the patient's arm was immobilized in a long arm cast for 6 weeks followed by 4 more weeks in a short arm cast (Figure 2). At the end of 10 weeks, the patient was started on protected activities with splint immobilization. Short-term fracture healing was uneventful, and alignment was maintained (Figure 3).

Current Problem and Treatment

The patient escaped follow-up and presented 4 years later with wrist deformity and pain with activities and writing. Physical examination demonstrated ulnar deviation of the wrist with full flexion and extension of the wrist. Subjectively the patient's strength was good; the neurovascular examination was also normal. Radiographs at this time showed ulnar shortening secondary to closure of the distal ulnar physis. The radius was longer than the ulna by 2 cm and was angulated ulnarly. The growth plate of the distal radius was open without apparent abnormality (Figure 4).

Discussion

Recognizing the Problem and Situations at High Risk

Inability to obtain and maintain reduction is a concern with metaphyseal fractures of the distal radius. Treatment of these fractures begins with attempted closed reduction using a combination of traction, angulation, and rotation of the palm in the direction of the angulation. Sustained longitudinal traction may be used with finger traps for completely displaced and bayoneted fractures. After the fracture is brought out to length, deformity exaggeration and rotation may produce end-to-end contact. It may be difficult to obtain apposition in completely displaced fractures because torn periosteum tightens around the

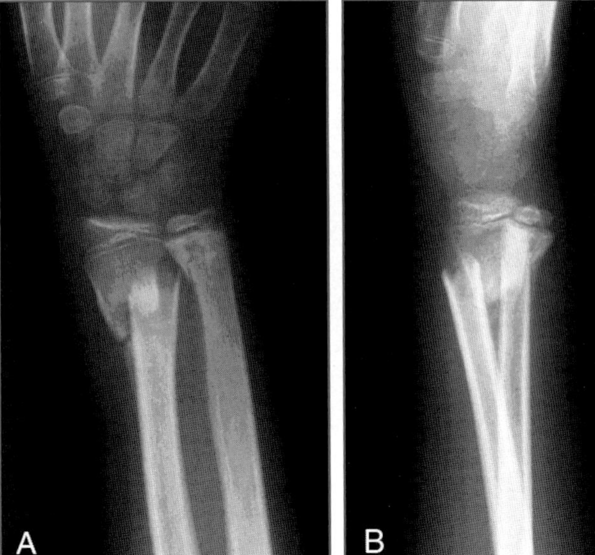

Figure 1 Example case: AP **(A)** and lateral **(B)** radiographs demonstrate a distal both-bone forearm fracture with 100% displacement of the radius. The ulnar fracture has definite extension into the physeal plate.

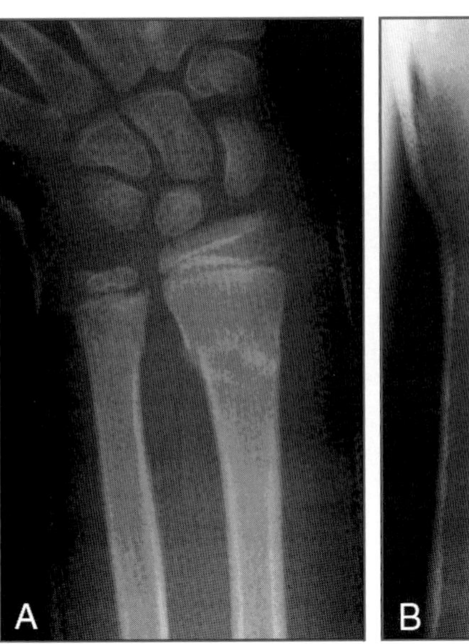

Figure 2 Example case: AP **(A)** and lateral **(B)** radiographs with the arm in a cast demonstrate excellent reduction of the ulna. Although the radius had 100% bayonet apposition, the reduction was accepted because of no angulation or loss in radial inclination.

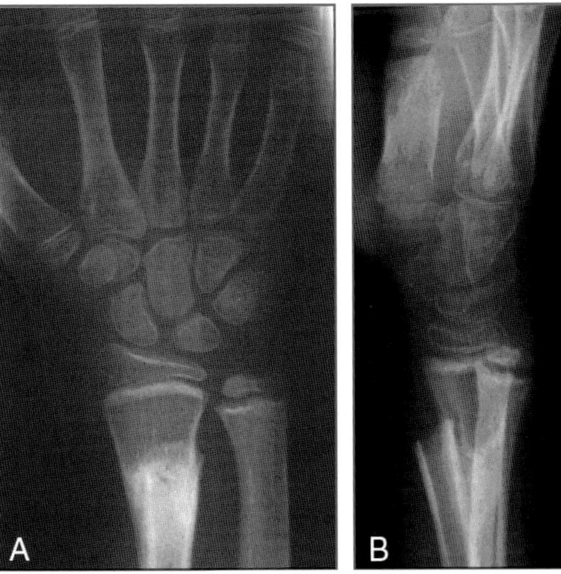

Figure 3 Example case: AP **(A)** and lateral **(B)** radiographs 3 months later demonstrate no change in alignment with exuberant dorsal callus.

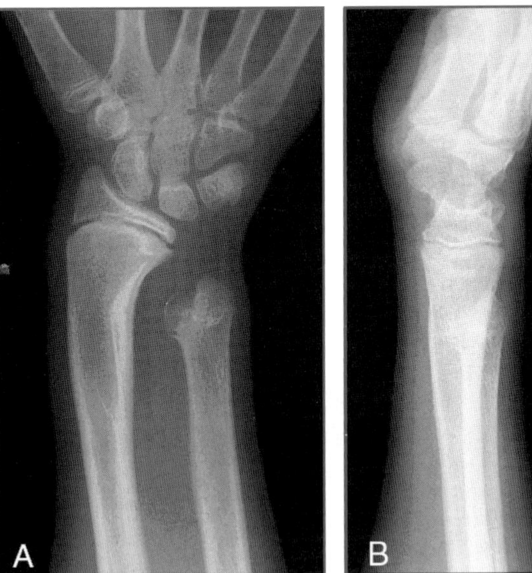

Figure 4 Example case: AP **(A)** and lateral **(B)** radiographs 4 years after the original injury. The ulna is shortened with apparent complete closure of the distal ulnar physis. The radial fracture is completely remodeled; however, ulnar deviation is present as a result of the ulnar shortening.

buttonholed proximal fragment.[1] Other common obstacles to reduction include the intact ulna, interposed periosteum or tendons, and fractures with reversed fracture obliquity. As described in the above case, it is acceptable to leave the fragments overlapped as long as rotation and angulation are maintained to less than 20° in children younger than age 12 years.[1]

A consensus of currently acceptable limits of displacement is reported in the literature, including bayonet apposition in children up to ages 10 to 12 years. Up to 20° of dorsal angulation is acceptable in children younger than ages 12 (girls) to 14 (boys) years; up to 15° of residual radial ulnar angulation is acceptable in girls up to age 12 years and in boys up to age 14.

Distal ulnar physeal fractures are uncommon (< 5% of radial fractures have an associated ulnar physeal fracture[2,3]) and may be difficult to diagnose because the secondary center of ossification usually does not appear radiographically prior to age 6 years.[2] In a review of physeal fractures, distal ulnar physeal fractures comprised 5.7% of all growth plate fractures.[4] Although most ulnar physeal injuries are associated with distal radial fractures, the relative rarity of physeal injuries may be a result of the apparent higher association of ulnar styloid fractures with distal radial fractures.[2]

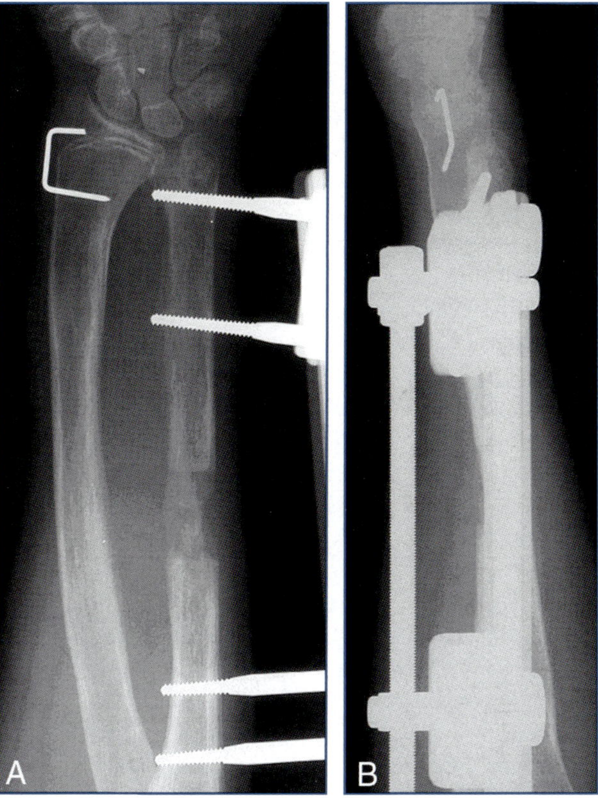

Figure 5 Example case: AP **(A)** and lateral **(B)** radiographs show the placement of the distal radial staple, which is designed to decrease ulnar inclination. The ulna has had an external fixator applied, osteotomy, and gradual lengthening of the midshaft of the ulna.

Management of Physeal Fractures

In cases of late displacement, manipulation can be repeated within 10 to 14 days after the fracture (Figure 5). Much beyond 2 weeks, the fracture is usually well healed and not amenable to such manipulation. In those instances, it is reasonable to observe a fracture malunion and perform an osteotomy at a later date should symptoms develop or remodeling appear inadequate. It is difficult to judge and predict eventual growth of each individual; therefore, I recommend observing a fracture malunion until the physis is closed before considering osteotomy.

Remanipulation may be helpful when angulation occurs in the early follow-up period. An alternative to remanipulation is preemptive single percutaneous pin fixation for fractures that are at risk for loss of reduction. In two randomized studies, percutaneous pinning was reported to decrease the need for remanipulation in distal radial fractures.[5,6] Although these studies and others suggest that closed reduction and percutaneous pinning prevents loss of reduction, there is currently no evidence that proves this approach has long-term clinical benefit compared to vigilant observation and appropriate remanipulation.[7] In the short term, routine percutaneous pinning of these fractures also has associated risks, including infection, hardware failure, and growth arrest.[8]

I believe that prophylactic pinning is almost never required because distal radial fractures remodel rapidly in children. If the child has 2 years of growth remaining, distal radial metaphyseal fractures will remodel complete displacement, 20° dorsal volar angulation, and 15° radial ulnar tilt.[1] The remodeling potential of the distal radius is so great that Do and associates[9] have recommended avoiding reduction of fractures that are less than 1 cm long and less than 15°

angulated in any direction. Immediate pinning may be prudent if an adolescent patient (who has little growth remaining) has an unstable fracture pattern. Selected patients may undergo closed reduction and percutaneous pinning with a Kirschner wire from the metaphysis to the epiphysis. Although it is always a good idea to avoid pinning across the physis if it all possible, growth arrest from pinning in uncomplicated fractures is uncommon.[10]

Treatment of an ulnar physeal fracture depends on the associated radial injury as well as the ulnar fracture. I recommend reduction of ulnar physeal fractures to within 2 mm of anatomicity. Difficulty in obtaining closed reduction may result from a tear in the joint capsule or interposition of the extensor carpi ulnaris tendon or periosteum.[11,12]

Ulnar physeal injuries are more likely to result in premature growth arrest than radial physeal injuries.[13] Golz and associates[2] reviewed 18 distal ulnar physeal fractures and reported premature growth arrest in 55%. From these data, they concluded that anatomic reduction is indicated but also admit that this rate may be reflective of the energy absorbed at injury and not the quality of reduction.[2]

Younger patients with ulnar arrest will have ulnar shortening (up to 4 cm), with resultant radial tethering and bowing of the diaphysis and ulnar deviation with altered mechanics of the wrist. It is rare for radial head subluxation to result from the discrepancy in the lengths of the ulna and radius. It has been noted that unacceptable cosmesis may be the most likely short-term result of ulnar shortening.[14] The long-term function and natural history of ulna minus forearms are currently unknown. For instance, there is a relationship between a shortened ulna and Kienböck's disease; however, a direct causal correlation has not been established.[15] Other disease processes such as multiple hereditary osteochondromatosis also exist, but an incidence of eventual wrist arthrosis is very rare.[16] Despite the lack of consistent evidence, I believe that having a shortened ulna leads to decreased rotation and, therefore, decreased function,[14] premature osteoarthrosis, or Kienböck's disease. Other indications for treatment include decreased range of motion, decreased grip strength, and unacceptable and progressive ulnar deviation of the hand.[17]

Treatment of premature ulnar arrest depends on the extent of physeal arrest, existing discrepancy, and growth remaining. Consideration for radial growth arrest would be reasonable in a patient with a known complete growth arrest of the ulna prior to progressive ulnar shortening. Physeal bar excision and fat interposition are not usually considered as treatment options, except in very young patients with a small bar (< 25%). However, in the upper extremity, it is probably more important to restore the radius-ulna relationship as opposed to restoring total limb length (as indicated in the lower extremity). The former can be accomplished with more reliable methods of radial shortening or ulnar lengthening and is preferable to the unpredictable results following bar excision. Other options include combinations of radial epiphysiodesis,[14] corrective osteotomy of the radius, gradual lengthening of the ulna, or acute lengthening of the ulna with bone grafting.[18]

Preventing the Problem

For unstable distal radial fractures, a long arm cast may help maintain the reduction, although Chess and associates[19] have suggested that a properly applied short arm cast will suffice. I tend to position dorsally displaced fractures in slight pronation even though recent evidence has suggested no relationship of hand position with reangulation.[20] I avoid fiberglass overwrapping because it does not allow for effective cast splitting in the immediate postfracture period. A single volar split in the plaster and slight spreading are recommended to accommodate swelling. In general, it is appropriate to univalve a cast on the side opposite the direction of likely displacement. This method allows some swelling yet maintains an intact surface to prevent displacement. Bivalving the cast or hospital admission is prudent if swelling is expected as a result of the severity of the fracture or of vigorous attempts at closed reduction. It is reasonable to admit a child if concerns for compartment syndrome remain or if unreliable care at home is likely.

Close follow-up is needed, with radiographs taken at 5 to 7 and 12 to 14 days after the fracture. This close monitoring is critical to detect repeat displacement and the need for further treatment. Relatively high rates of reangulation (from 11% to 62.5%) have been reported in isolated distal radial fractures.[1,5,21-25] Higher rates of reangulation are noted in fractures with apex volar angulation and complete fractures than in greenstick fractures.[25] In general, the

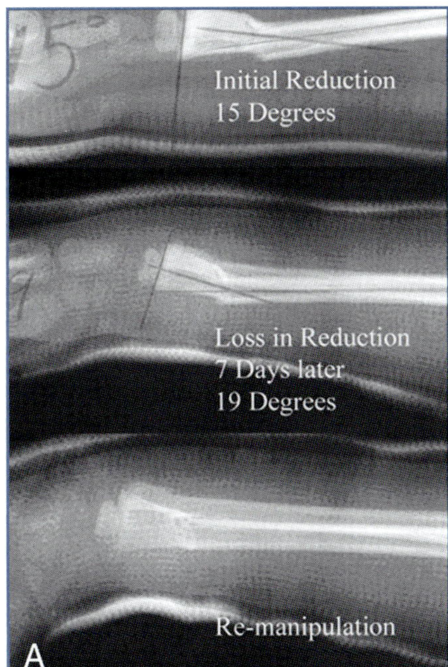

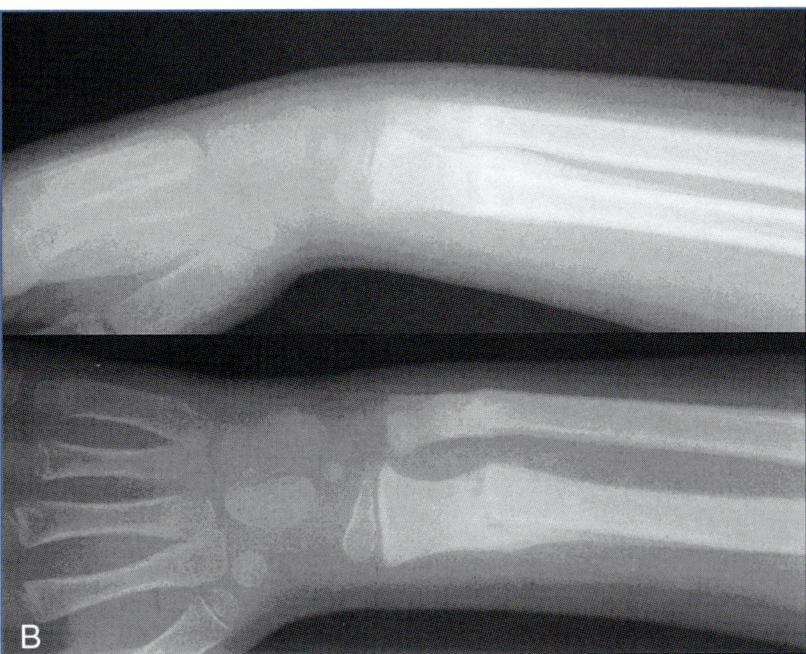

Figure 6 A, A 6-year-old girl with a distal both-bone fracture was treated with cast immobilization without reduction. At 7 days' follow-up, the fracture was displaced to 19°; gentle molding with volar flexion and application of a better cast restored acceptable alignment in the office. **B,** At 5 weeks, the fracture healed in the reduced position. No additional problems have developed, and the fracture has fully recovered with no deficits.

most important risk factors for reangulation during immobilization in the immediate postfracture period are degree of initial displacemen[5] and quality of the initial reduction.[24] Several investigators have reported that fractures with more than 50% translation tended to require further treatment.[1,23]

Physeal fractures resulting in premature ulnar arrest are rare because ulnar physeal fractures are rare. Ray and associates[17] reviewed a total of 28 cases combined from their experience and from the literature. Even though this complication is rare, individuals with physeal fractures should be followed closely in an attempt to detect premature closure of the physis and subsequent deformities. Radiographs will first detect physeal arrest at 6 months after injury. Comparison to contralateral wrist radiographs is indicated with time to document premature arrest. Ray and associates[17] developed a classification system of ulnar arrest patterns, yet the clinical significance of this system is not known.

Case Management and Outcome Summary

After appropriate preoperative counseling, the patient underwent distal radial hemiepiphyseal stapling and ulnar lengthening. Surgery was performed uneventfully, and the patient was discharged to home. He returned 10 days later and distraction was begun at 1 mm per day until 2 cm of length was attained. The patient had excellent callus formation (Figure 6), and after full maturation of the regenerated bone, the device was removed 5 months after the original surgery. The patient's arm was immobilized in a splint for several weeks, and he was allowed to gradually increase activities. Two months after the fixator was removed, he had full range of motion with slight tenosynovitis over the dorsal radial aspect of the radius. With time, the activity-related pain that was noted preoperatively

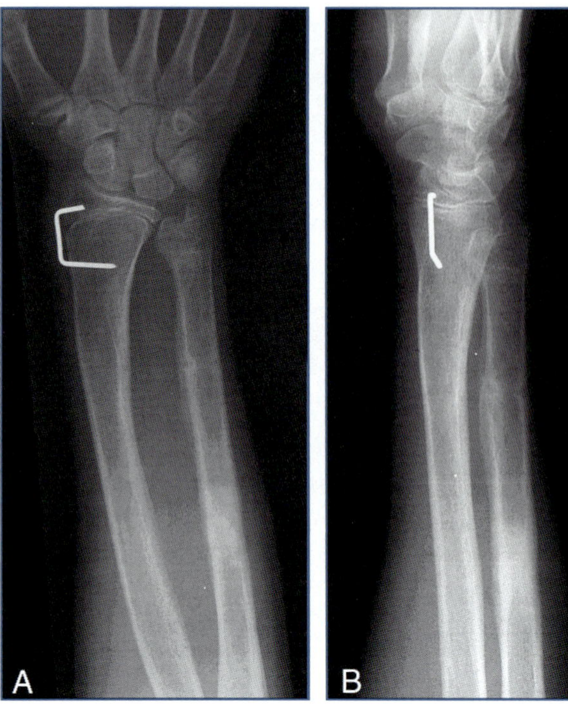

Figure 7 Example case: Final AP **(A)** and lateral **(B)** radiographs demonstrate full healing of the ulna. Residual ulnar deviation of the radius is present despite the presence of the staple. Further growth and remodeling will be expected until maturity.

had resolved. The final radiographs demonstrated excellent healing and good alignment (Figure 7).

Strategies to Minimize Common Complications

Distal radius fractures are common, and a large amount of displacement can be accepted. In general, 20° of dorsal displacement and complete bayonet apposition is acceptable in girls to age 12 years and boys to age 14 years. The potential for fracture reangulation and subsequent malunion may exist in up to one third of patients with significantly displaced fractures with less than anatomic reduction. Early follow-up and remanipulation are recommended should loss in reduction occur. Consideration of preemptive, percutaneous pinning of isolated distal radius fracture is reasonable in patients with little growth remaining because higher rates of repeat displacement exist with little chance for remodeling due to age. Distal ulnar physeal fractures are rare; however, the incidence of growth arrest is not, and patients should be followed carefully.

Clinical problems in the current case included gradual increase in pain and ulnar deviation of the wrist. Reconstruction was recommended because the patient had symptoms. Ulnar lengthening was performed gradually in addition to radial hemiepiphyseal stapling. Final follow-up is pending but continued gradual improvement in radial inclination is expected.

Acknowledgments

I would like to thank Mark Birnbaum, MD, Orlando, Florida, for allowing me to use the above case for this publication.

References

1. Roy DR: Completely displaced distal radius fractures with intact ulnas in children. *Orthopedics* 1989; 12:1089-1092.
2. Golz RJ, Grogan DP, Greene TL, Belsole RJ, Ogden JA: Distal ulnar physeal injury. *J Pediatr Orthop* 1991;11:318-326.
3. Walsh HP, McLaren CA, Owen R: Galeazzi fractures in children. *J Bone Joint Surg Br* 1987;69: 730-733.
4. Peterson CA, Peterson HA: Analysis of the incidence of injuries to the epiphyseal growth plate. *J Trauma* 1972;12:275-281.
5. McLauchlan GJ, Cowan B, Annan IH, Robb JE: Management of completely displaced metaphyseal fractures of the distal radius in children. *J Bone Joint Surg Br* 2002;84: 413-417.
6. Gibbons CL, Woods DA, Pailthorpe C, Carr AJ, Worlock P: The management of isolated distal radius fractures in children. *J Pediatr Orthop* 1994;14:207-210.

7. Price CT: Management of completely displaced metaphyseal fractures of the distal radius in children. *J Bone Joint Surg Am* 2002;84: 2109.
8. Boyden MP, Peterson HA: Partial premature closure of the distal radial physis associated with Kirschner wire fixation. *Orthopedics* 1994;14: 507-508.
9. Do TT, Strub WM, Ford SL, Mehlman CT, Crawford AH: Reduction versus remodeling in pediatric distal forearm fractures: A preliminary cost analysis. *J Pediatr Orthop* 2003;12:111-115.
10. Choi KY, Chan WS, Lam TP, Cheng JC: Percutaneous Kirschner pinning for severely displaced distal radial fractures in children: A report of 157 cases. *J Bone Joint Surg Br* 1995;77:797-801.
11. Engber WD, Keene JS: Irreducible fracture separation of the distal ulnar epiphysis: Report of a case. *J Bone Joint Surg Am* 1985;67: 1130-1132.
12. Evans DL, Stauber M, Frykman GK: Irreducible epiphyseal plate fracture of the distal ulna due to interposition of the extensor carpi ulnaris tendon. *Clin Orthop* 1990; 251:162-165.
13. Lipschultz O: The end-results of injuries to the epiphysis. *Radiology* 1937;28:223-232.
14. Nelson OA, Buchanan JR, Harrison CS: Distal ulnar growth arrest. *J Hand Surg [Am]* 1984;9:164-171.
15. Nathan PA, Meadows KD: Ulnaminus variance and Kienbock's disease. *J Hand Surg [Am]* 1987;12: 777-778.
16. Noonan KJ, Levenda A, Snead JW, Feinberg JR, Mih AD: The natural history of multiple hereditary osteochondromatosis (MHO): Functional outcome and implications for treatment in children. *J Bone Joint Surg Am* 2002;84:397-403.
17. Ray TD, Tessler RH, Dell PC: Traumatic ulnar physeal arrest after distal forearm fractures in children. *J Pediatr Orthop* 1996;16:195-200.
18. Waters PM, Van Heest AE, Emans J: Acute forearm lengthenings. *J Pediatr Orthop* 1997;17:444-449.
19. Chess DG, Hyndman JC, Leahey JL, Brown DCS, Sinclair AM: Short arm plaster cast for distal pediatric forearm fractures. *J Pediatr Orthop* 1994;14:211-213.
20. Boyer BA, Overton B, Schrader W, Riley P, Fleissner P: Position of immobilization for pediatric forearm fractures. *J Pediatr Orthop* 2002;22: 185-187.
21. Davis DR, Green DP: Forearm fractures in children: Pitfalls and complications. *Clin Orthop* 1976;120: 172-184.
22. Green JS, Williams SC, Finlay D, Harper WM: Distal forearm fractures in children: The role of radiographs during follow-up. *Injury* 1998;29:309-312.
23. Mani GV, Hui PW, Cheng JCY: Translation of the radius as a predictor of outcome in distal radial fractures of children. *J Bone Joint Surg Br* 1993;75:808-811.
24. Proctor MT, Moore DJ, Patterson JMH: Redisplacement after manipulation of distal radial fractures in children. *J Bone Joint Surg Br* 1993;75:453-454.
25. Schranz PJ, Fagg PS: Undisplaced fractures of the distal third of the radius in children: An innocent fracture? *Injury* 1992;23:165-167.

Chapter 3

Malunited Forearm Fractures

Charles T. Price, MD

Case Presentation

History

A 9-year, 9-month-old girl sustained a severely angulated midshaft fracture of the radius and ulna when she slipped off a low wall (Figure 1). Closed reduction and cast immobilization maintained satisfactory alignment (Figure 2). Six weeks after the initial injury, the cast was removed, and she was allowed to return to light activities (Figure 3).

Current Problem and Treatment

Three months after the initial injury and 6 weeks after cast removal, she fell again and refractured her forearm in the same location (Figure 4). Treatment of the second fracture consisted of closed reduction and cast immobilization (Figure 5).

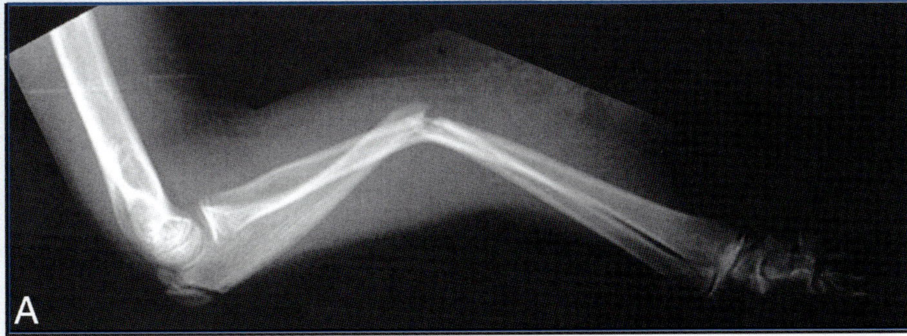

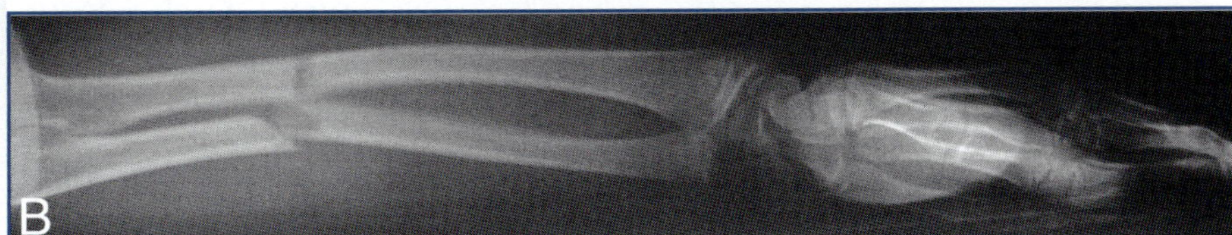

Figure 1 Example case: AP **(A)** and lateral **(B)** radiographs of a 9-year, 9-month-old girl showing midshaft forearm fractures sustained when she slipped off a low wall.

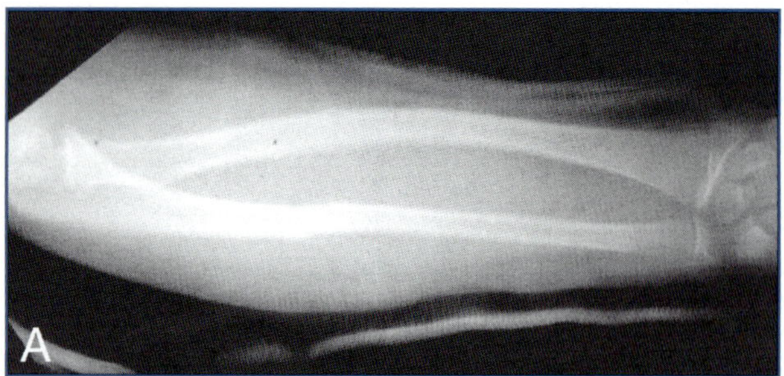

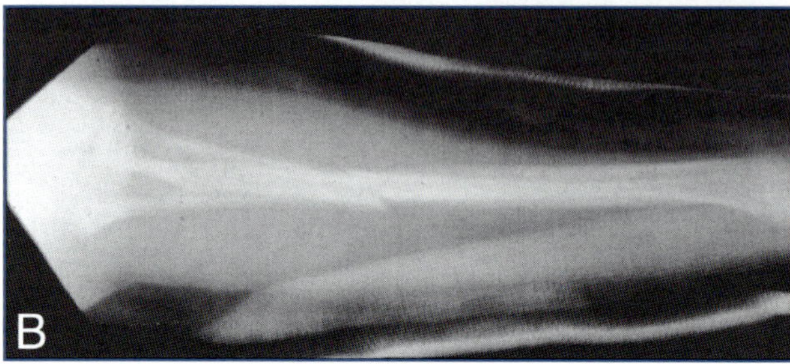

Figure 2 Example case: AP **(A)** and lateral **(B)** radiographs following closed reduction.

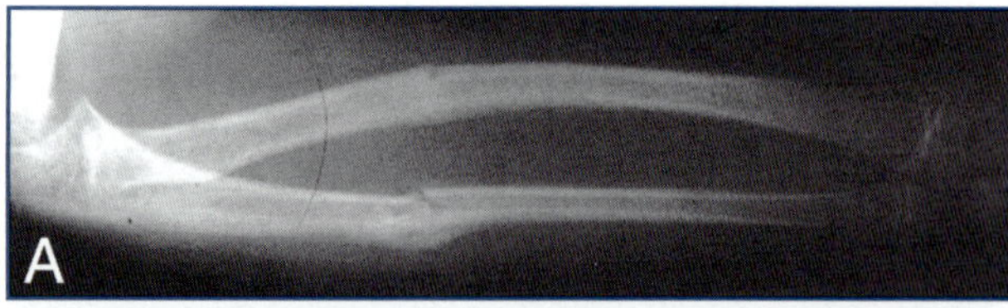

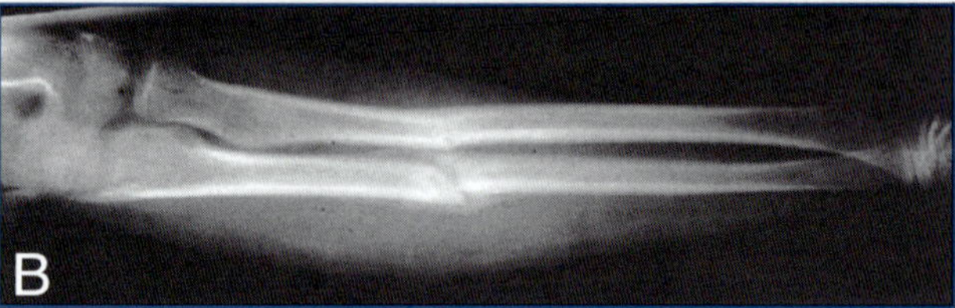

Figure 3 Example case: AP **(A)** and lateral **(B)** radiographs at the time of cast removal demonstrate callus formation and satisfactory alignment.

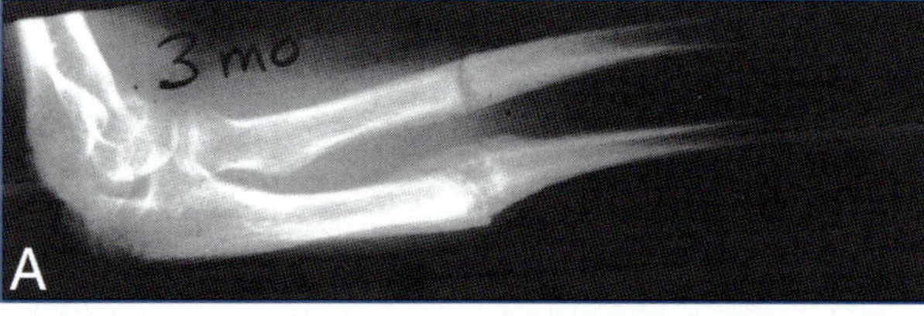

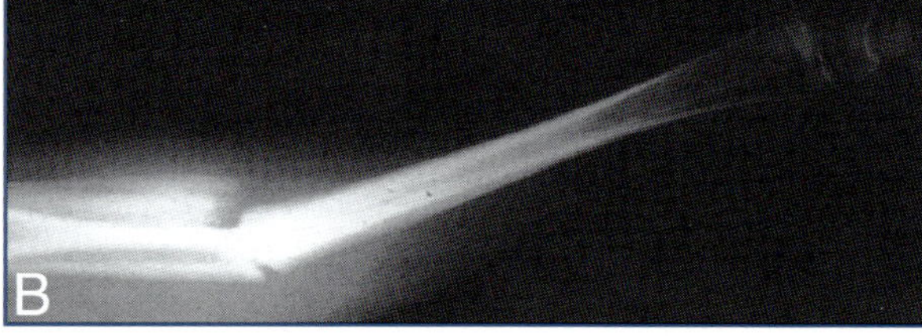

Figure 4 Example case: AP **(A)** and lateral **(B)** radiographs showing refracture of the forearm that occurred as a result of a fall 3 months after the initial injury.

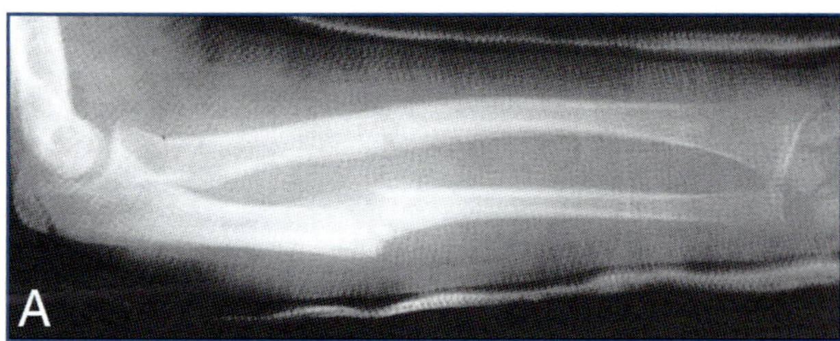

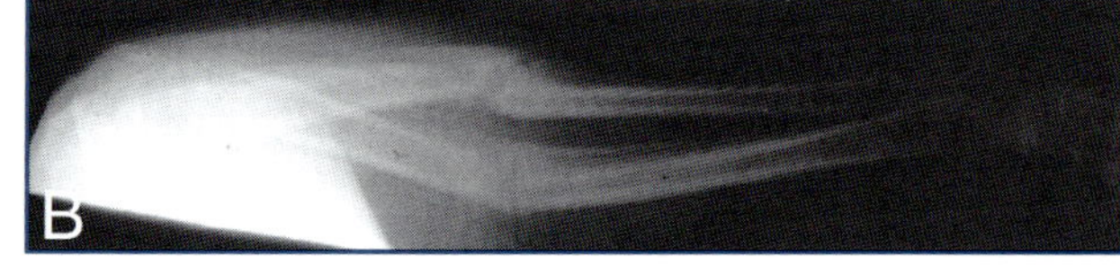

Figure 5 Example case: AP **(A)** and lateral **(B)** radiographs obtained after an attempted closed reduction following refracture demonstrate incomplete reduction.

Discussion

Recognizing Fractures at Risk for Malunion

Most forearm fractures in children can be managed by closed methods. However, certain fractures are more troublesome than others. Severely displaced forearm fractures in children may be difficult to reduce and maintain by cast immobilization alone. Despite adequate initial reduction, unstable fractures may lose reduction in a cast during the first 3 weeks after injury. Proximal forearm fractures are especially prone to unacceptable results with closed management.[1] Closed management of proximal forearm fractures may be facilitated by immobilization with the elbow in extension.[2] The thumb should be incorporated in the cast to prevent slippage. Careful attention to alignment is recommended in all forearm fractures. Complete displacement is acceptable, but angulation greater than 10° during early fracture healing may lead to poor results.[1] Wedging of the cast or gentle remolding without sedation during closed management can improve alignment without resorting to surgical intervention. However, surgical stabilization is recommended when adequate reduction cannot be obtained or maintained.

A refracture that displaces may be difficult to reduce and maintain in a reduced position as indicated in the case presentation. Refratures also unite slowly and may necessitate prolonged cast immobilization, increasing the risk of stiffness. Some refractures can be managed without surgical intervention, but open reduction with internal fixation may be preferred to facilitate anatomic alignment and early motion.[3,4] Greenstick fractures of the forearm shaft have the greatest risk of refracture. This risk has been attributed to the stability provided by the intact cortex that inhibits callus formation and leads to delayed union of the disrupted cortex. Fracturing the intact cortex during reduction or immobilization for a minimum of 6 weeks can reduce the risk of refracture when treating greenstick fractures of the forearm.[4,5]

Open reduction with internal fixation should be considered for initial management of refractures with displacement, open fractures, displaced fractures of the proximal forearm, unstable fractures, or unacceptable alignment following attempted closed reduction.[1,3,6-8] Surgical stabilization may also facilitate the management of high-energy forearm fractures, such as segmental fractures, and floating elbow injuries.

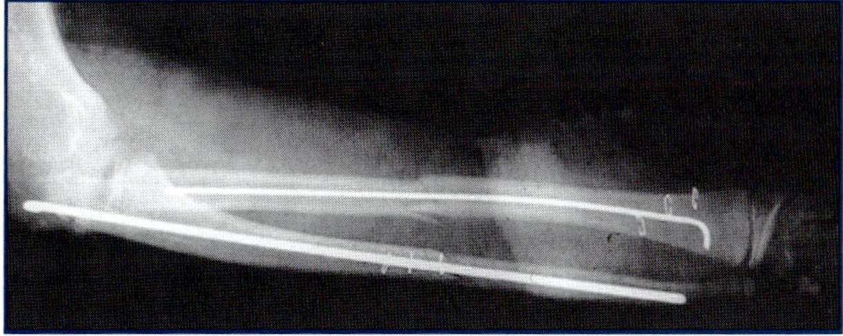

Figure 6 Flexible IM nails provide satisfactory fixation for most pediatric and adolescent forearm fractures.

Preventing Malunion

Surgical stabilization for pediatric and adolescent forearm fractures can be achieved by flexible intramedullary (IM) fixation (Figure 6). This technique is relatively simple, minimally invasive, and generally produces excellent results. Supplemental cast immo-

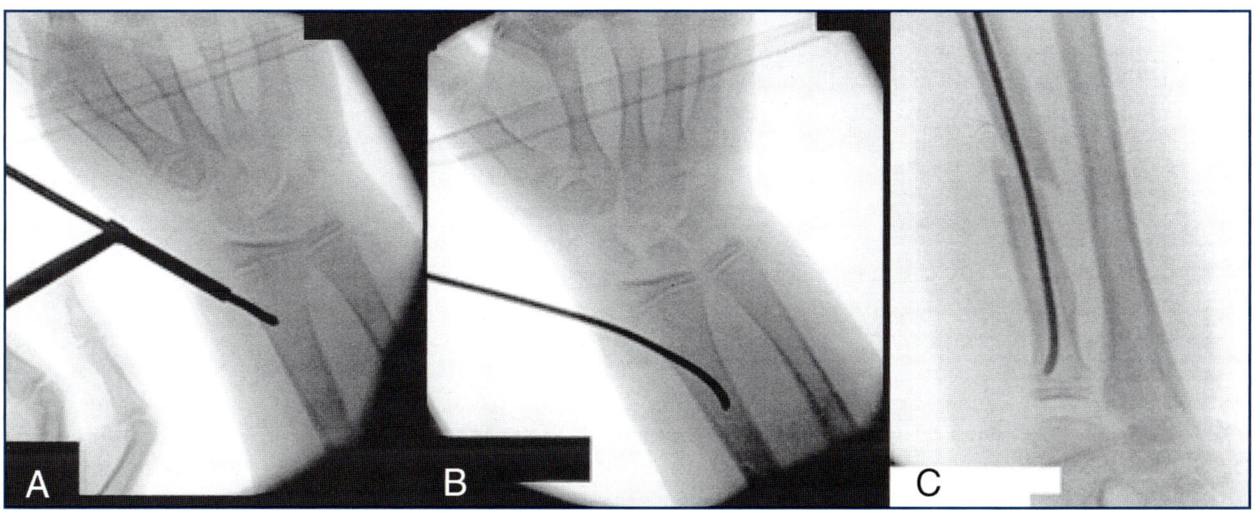

Figure 7 Technique for inserting a flexible IM nail into the radius. **A,** An oblique drill hole is made in the distal radial metaphysis. Care is taken to avoid drilling the opposite cortex in order to avoid creating a pocket that could trap the tip of the flexible nail or pin. **B,** A flexible Steinmann pin or titanium nail is passed into the IM canal of the radius. **C,** The nail or pin is passed across the fracture site. Anatomic reduction is not required as long as alignment can be maintained.

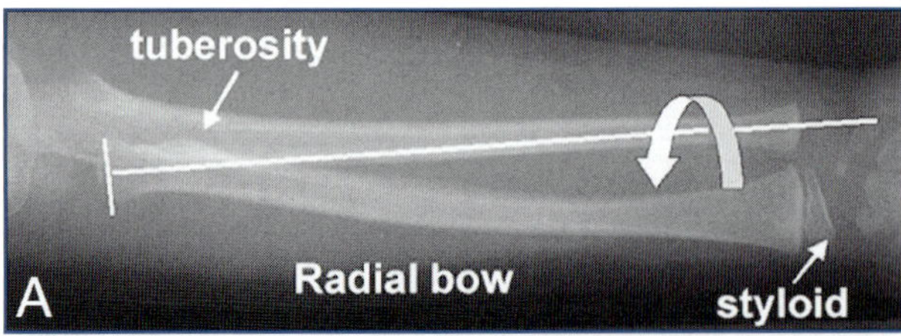

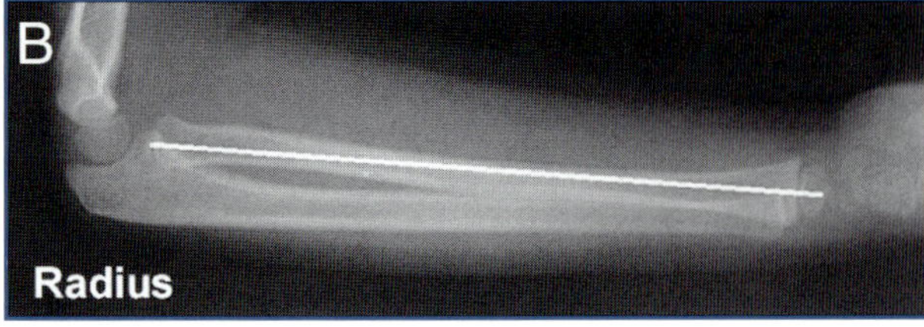

Figure 8 AP **(A)** and lateral **(B)** views showing the normal anatomic landmarks of the radius. Note that the radial bow is directed laterally in the midshaft. The tuberosity of the radius and styloid are approximately on opposite sides of the bone.

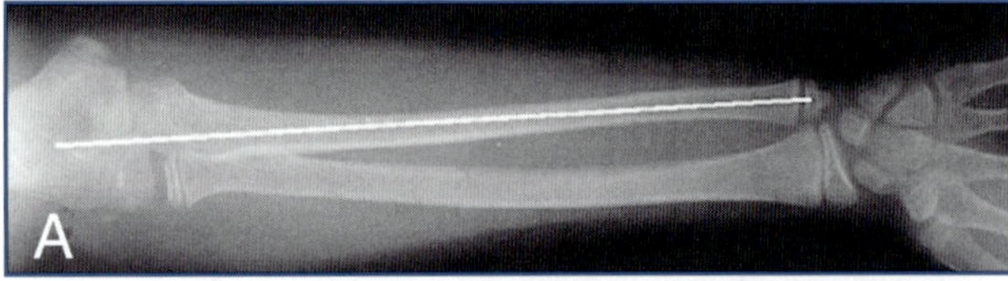

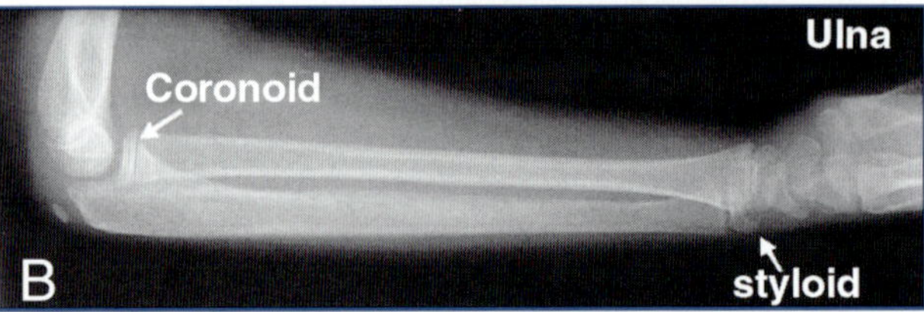

Figure 9 AP **(A)** and lateral **(B)** views showing the normal anatomic landmarks of the ulna. Note that the ulna has a slight varus angulation proximally and is essentially straight in the lateral view.

bilization for 6 weeks can facilitate maintenance of reduction. Six weeks of immobilization is unlikely to affect motion in children, and nonunion is uncommon in children. For these reasons IM fixation is preferred; rigid internal fixation with plates and screws is rarely necessary.[9]

The technique for IM nailing of pediatric forearm fractures has been well described in textbooks and other publications.[10,11] I prefer to stabilize the ulna with an IM nail introduced proximally, just lateral to the tip of the olecranon. This nail may be a small Rush rod, a Steinmann pin, or an elastic titanium nail. After the ulna is stabilized, then a flexible Steinmann pin (0.062-in) or titanium nail is introduced into the radius from the distal metaphysis (Figure 7). One or two attempts are made to pass the nails with closed manipulation, but a small exposure for open reduction is preferred to multiple failed attempts at closed nailing. Tourniquet time should be kept to a minimum and should not exceed 1 hour. The risk of forearm compartment syndrome may be increased by multiple failed attempts at closed pinning and prolonged tourniquet time.

Management of Malunion

Occasionally, malunion occurs regardless of the method of management. In these instances, the surgeon must decide whether correction of the deformity should be recommended. The indications for correction of malunited forearm fractures have not been clearly defined. Remodeling can be expected to improve cosmesis in moderate forearm malunion; however, the principal functional concern is loss of forearm rotation. Because most daily activities can be accomplished with 50° of pronation and 50° of supination,[12] some loss of forearm rotation is acceptable. In cadaver studies, significant loss of forearm rotation has been noted when angular deformity in the midshaft is 15° to 20°.[13,14] Therefore, I believe that angular deformity of less than 20° can be accepted in most cases of pediatric and adolescent forearm fracture malunion.

Remodeling and compensatory shoulder or wrist movement can be expected to produce a satisfactory result for malunion measuring less than 20°. Angulation of 20° to 30° may or may not improve to allow recovery of motion with acceptable cosmesis. Distal forearm deformity is less likely to restrict movement than proximal forearm deformity.[1,13] Two to 3 months of observation may be useful for malunion of 20° to 30°. If deformity is still unacceptable or motion is limited after 2 to 3 months of observation, then corrective osteotomy is indicated. Trousdale and Linscheid[15] reported that more motion is restored when an osteotomy is performed within the first year following the initial injury. When the angulation is greater than 30°, early osteotomy is indicated because adequate remodeling and restoration of motion is less likely.

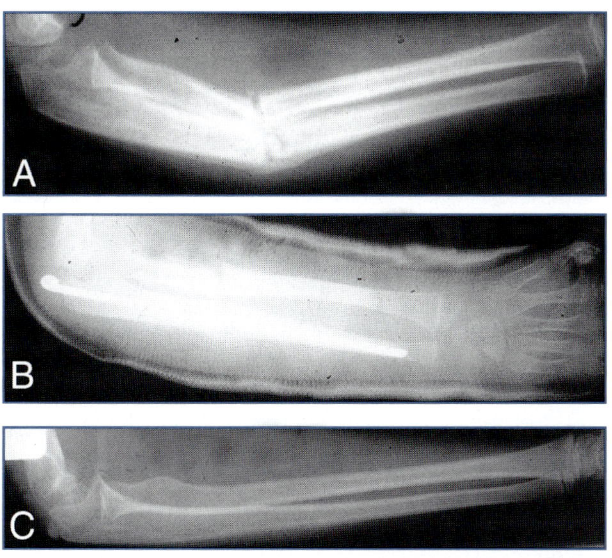

Figure 10 A, A 5-year-old girl with a 30° malunion of the proximal radius and ulna. Early correction of the deformity is recommended for malunion of 30° or greater in any plane. **B,** Osteotomies of the radius and ulna were performed. A Rush rod in the ulna is often sufficient immobilization in younger children. Lateral **(C)** and AP **(D)** radiographs obtained at long-term follow-up demonstrate excellent alignment. The patient recovered full range of motion.

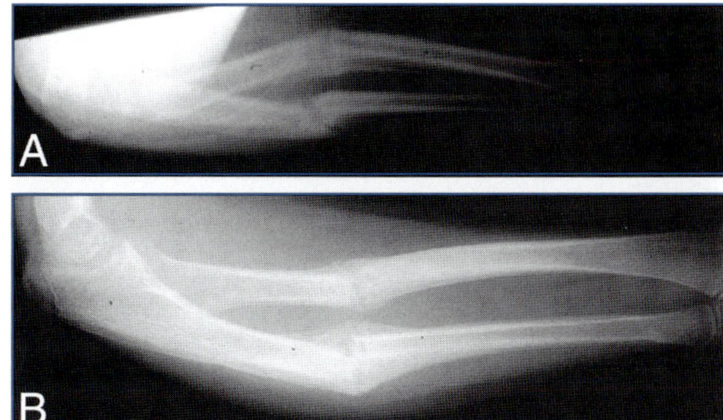

Figure 11 Example case: Lateral **(A)** and AP **(B)** radiographs showing delayed union with deterioration of alignment in cast immobilization.

When planning an osteotomy for correction of malunion, it is important to understand the anatomic shape of the radius and ulna. Figures 8 and 9 show the normal anatomy of these two bones. Note that the radial bow is directed laterally in the midshaft while the radial tuberosity and styloid are on approximately opposite sides of the bone. The ulna has a slight varus angulation proximally and is essentially straight in the lateral projection. The ulnar styloid is on the opposite side of the bone from the coronoid process.

For children younger than age 8 years, the osteotomy may be stabilized with intramedullary fixation of one or both bones (Figure 10). However, I recommend fixation with plates and screws in older children to allow for early stable motion. The technique involves exposing both bones through separate incisions. The ulna is approached along its subcutaneous border, and the radius is exposed through the anterior Henry approach. Following exposure of each bone, the osteotomies are performed at the malunion site and in the position of maximum deformity as determined by intraoperative imaging. Intraoperative fluoroscopy allows determination of the maximum apex of deformity. Perpendicular V-shaped osteotomy is then performed at the apex. Then the ulna is stabilized in the corrected alignment, followed by stabilization of the radius in the corrected alignment. It may be necessary to shorten one bone slightly to allow bone-to-bone apposition of both osteotomy sites. Bone grafting is rarely necessary in children and adolescents. Postoperative management consists of a bivalved cast or splint for 24 to 72 hours followed by a long arm cast for up to 6 weeks.

Case Management and Outcome Summary

When the cast was removed 6 weeks after the refracture, deformity and malunion were apparent. The forearm was in neutral position and regained only 40° of forearm rotation after 6 weeks (Figure 11). Osteotomy was performed, restoring alignment and a radial bow. A Rush rod was used to stabilize the ulna and a one-third tubular plate was used to secure the radius (Figure 12). One year after the osteotomy, full

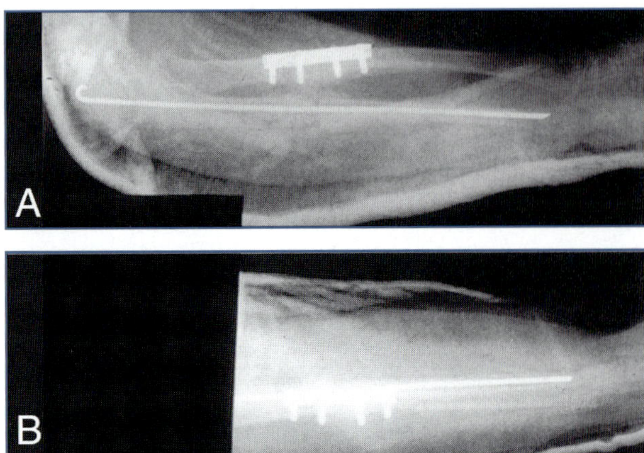

Figure 12 Example case: AP **(A)** and lateral **(B)** radiographs 7 months after the initial injury demonstrating that an osteotomy was performed with a Rush rod in the ulna and rigid fixation of the radius.

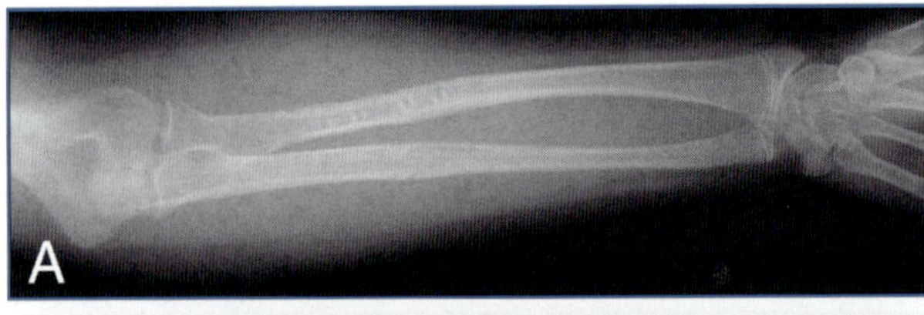

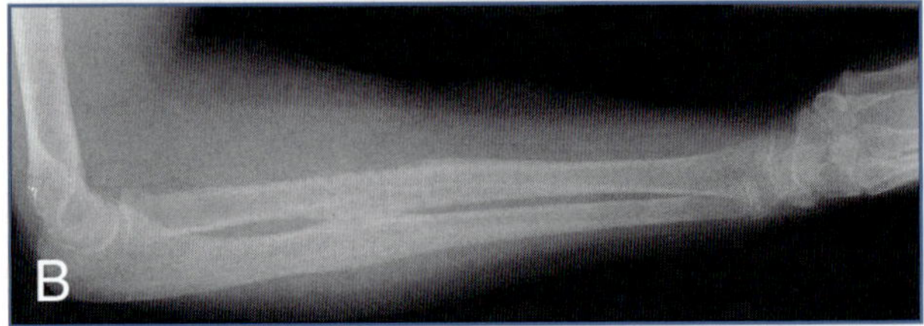

Figure 13 Example case: AP **(A)** and lateral **(B)** radiographs obtained after removal of internal fixation. Note that normal alignment was restored, and the patient recovered full range of motion.

range of motion was restored and the implants were removed (Figure 13).

Strategies to Minimize Common Complications

Malunited forearm fractures in children may occur despite proper management. In the case described in this chapter, open reduction with internal fixation should have been performed at the time of the refracture because it would have avoided malunion. However, subsequent osteotomy was performed a few weeks after malunion was recognized. The final outcome was satisfactory because normal alignment was restored.

Midshaft malunion of less than 20° may be acceptable, but osteotomy is recommended for malunion greater than 30°. Malunion is more likely to occur following reduction of severely displaced forearm fractures, proximal fractures, and refractures than in greenstick and stable fractures. Most forearm fractures can be managed by closed methods, but flexible IM nailing should be considered when closed methods are unsuccessful. Correction of malunion is best performed within 1 year of injury.

Acknowledgment

I would like to thank Raymond Knapp, MD, of Orlando, Florida, for allowing publication of the illustrative case at the beginning of this chapter.

References

1. Price CT, Scott DS, Kurzner ME, Flynn JC: Malunited forearm fractures in children. *J Pediatr Orthop* 1990;10:705-712.
2. Walker JL, Rang M: Forearm fractures in children: Cast treatment with the elbow extended. *J Bone Joint Surg Br* 1991;73:299-301.
3. Arunachalam VS, Griffiths JC: Fracture recurrence in children. *Injury* 1975;7:37-40.
4. Schwartz N, Pienaar S, Schwarz AF, Jelen M, Styhler W, Jayr J: Refracture of the forearm in children. *J Bone Joint Surg Br* 1996;78:740-744.
5. Bould M, Bannister GC: Refractures of the radius and ulna in children. *Injury* 1999;30:583-586.
6. Greenbaum B, Zionts LE, Ebramzadeh E: Open fractures of the forearm in children. *J Orthop Trauma* 2001;15:111-118.
7. Haasbeek JF, Cole WG: Open fractures of the arm in children. *J Bone Joint Surg Br* 1995;77:576-581.
8. Thompson GH, Wilber JH, Marcus RE: Internal fixation of fractures in

children and adolescents. *Clin Orthop* 1984;188:10-20.

9. Van der Reis WL, Otsuka NY, Moroz P, Mah J: Intramedullary nailing versus plate fixation for unstable forearm fractures in children. *J Pediatr Orthop* 1998;18: 9-13.
10. Lascombes P, Prevot MD, Ligier JN, Metaizeau JP, Poncelet T: Elastic stable intramedullary nailing of forearm shaft fractures in children: 85 cases. *J Pediatr Orthop* 1990;10:167-171.
11. Smith H, Sage FP: Medullary fixation of forearm fractures. *J Bone Joint Surg Am* 1957;39:91-98.
12. Morrey BF, Askew LJ, Chao EY: A biomechanical study of normal functional elbow motion. *J Bone Joint Surg Am* 1981;63:872-877.
13. Tarr RR, Garfinkel AI, Sarmiento A: The effects of angular and rotational deformities of both bones of the forearm. *J Bone Joint Surg Am* 1984;66:65-70.
14. Matthews LS, Kaufer H, Garver DF, Sonstegard DA: The effect on supination-pronation of angular malalignment of fractures of both bones of the forearm: An experimental study. *J Bone Joint Surg Am* 1982; 64:14-17.
15. Trousdale RT, Linscheid RL: Operative treatment of malunited fractures of the forearm. *J Bone Joint Surg Am* 1995;77:894-902.

Chapter 4

Monteggia Fracture Malunion

Peter M. Waters, MD

Case Presentation

History

A 7-year-old girl who fell on an extended arm on the playground 6 weeks ago had immediate pain and restricted motion in her forearm, wrist, and elbow. She was taken to the local emergency department where radiographs showed that she had an isolated ulnar fracture. Her arm was placed in a protective splint until the swelling decreased, and her parents were referred to an orthopaedist.

Examination 5 days later revealed less forearm swelling and a normal distal neurovascular examination. Repeat radiographs showed no change in the alignment of her ulnar fracture, which was deemed to be acceptable. She was placed in a long arm cast, and her parents were instructed to bring her back in 4 weeks for a cast change. At the time of her next follow-up, no radiographs were obtained, and her long arm cast was changed to a short arm cast.

At 6 weeks after the injury, her orthopaedist was alarmed to note that her radiographs showed a dislocated radial head (Figure 1). In reviewing her previous radiographs, he was further disturbed to note that he had not appreciated the original displacement of the radial head, which was now more obvious on the radiographs. After immediate consultation, the patient was referred to a pediatric hand surgeon.

Current Problem and Treatment

On urgent evaluation, the patient was noted to have palpable callus over the ulnar fracture and only minimal discomfort to palpation and percussion. Her dislocated radial head was palpable in the cubital fossa. Radial nerve function was intact, but she reported discomfort with palpation of the radial tunnel.

Discussion

Recognizing Monteggia Fracture-Dislocations

Treatment of Monteggia fracture-dislocations in children can be fraught with complications. The first major problem, which occurs far too often in these fractures, is the failure to recognize radiocapitellar subluxation or dislocation in the acute setting. Despite the common knowledge that the radiocapitellar joint

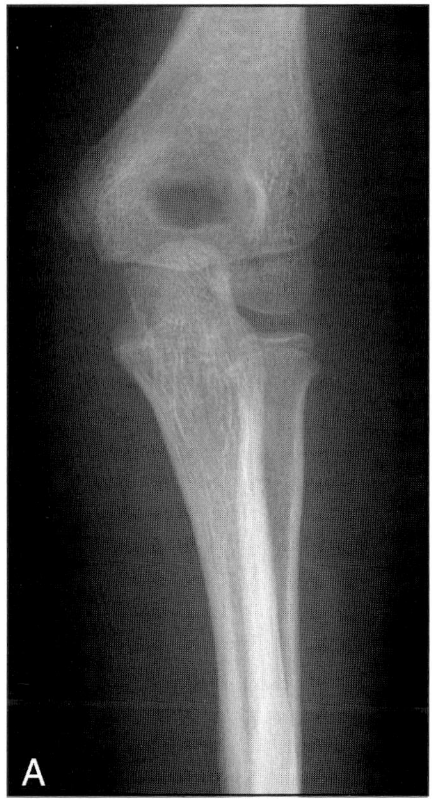

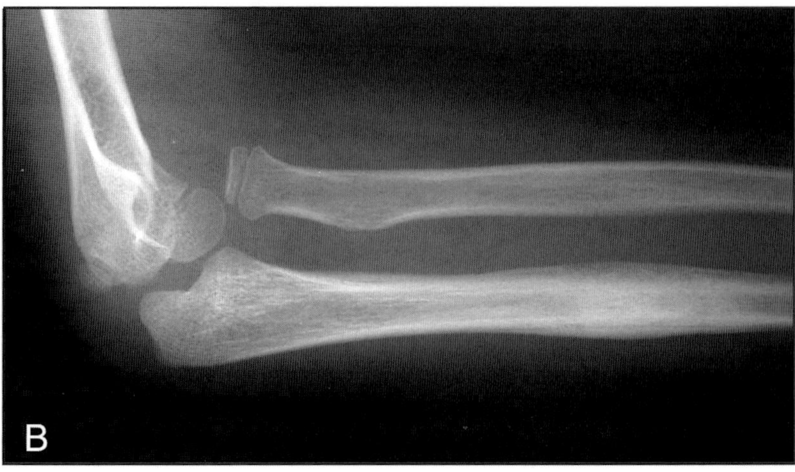

Figure 1 Example case: Preoperative AP **(A)** and lateral **(B)** radiographs of a healed ulnar fracture malunion and chronic radial head dislocation noted at 6 weeks postinjury.

must be anatomically aligned on all radiographic views,[1-5] Monteggia lesions continue to be missed with clinical consequences.[1,4-9] Restoring and maintaining anatomic alignment is much easier in the acute setting than with reconstruction of a chronic ulnar fracture malunion and radial head dislocation. Therefore, it is imperative that radiographs of all acute elbow and forearm injuries be examined closely for a Monteggia fracture-dislocation.

Management of Monteggia Fracture-Dislocations

Monteggia fracture-dislocations can be unstable and become displaced after closed reduction in children.[6,10,11] Internal fixation may be necessary to stabilize the reduction. The type of forearm fracture often guides the surgeon to the degree of postreduction stability. Plastic deformation and greenstick fractures are generally stable after closed reduction and can be treated in a long arm cast. Short oblique and transverse ulnar fractures should be treated with intramedullary (IM) fixation (Figure 2). Long oblique and comminuted fractures often require plate and screw fixation to maintain radial head reduction. Reducing and stabilizing the ulnar fracture is usually the key to preventing late loss of reduction in pediatric Monteggia lesions.[10,11]

On rare occasions, there is an isolated radial head dislocation, or the radial head does not reduce anatomically with reduction of the ulnar fracture. In these situations, open reduction of the radial head is indicated.[12-15] The annular ligament is often displaced and entrapped in the joint with dislocation of the radial head anteriorly through the capsule. The posterior interosseous nerve needs to be protected during surgical exposure and repair. An extended posterolateral incision and arthrotomy are used. In these situations in children, the annular ligament often separates from the ulnar periosteum intact and displaces over the radial head into the joint. The ligament can be mobilized to its anatomic location on the radial neck

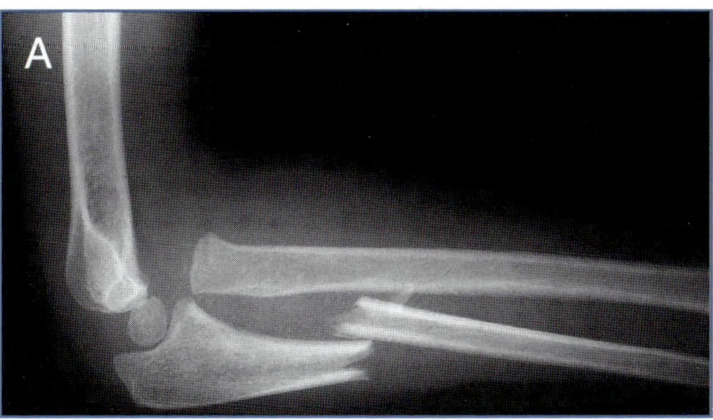

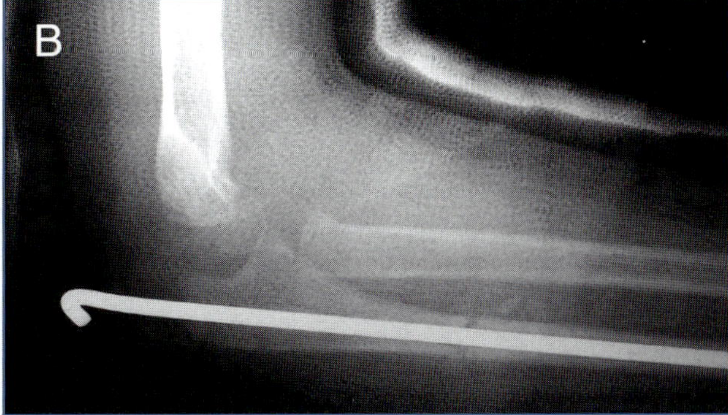

Figure 2 An acute Monteggia lesion with a transverse fracture of the ulna **(A)** treated with closed reduction and IM fixation **(B)**.

and the radial head reduced. The annular ligament is reattached with suture to the proximal ulna for stabilization.

Chronic Monteggia reconstruction is a more difficult surgical endeavor. There are historic publications that advocate leaving the malunion and dislocation alone,[16-18] with consideration for late radial head excision if symptoms warrant. Most authors, however, are concerned about loss of motion and function, osteoarthritis and pain, and progressive valgus deformity with a chronic Monteggia lesion in young children.[8,9,19-25] Multiple small, retrospective case series have been reported with different techniques and results that range from excellent to disastrous (Figure 3). Techniques advocated have included annular ligament reconstruction alone (with native ligament, regional fascia or tendons, and free grafts); osteotomy alone (with no fixation, internal and external fixation); and combined osteotomy and annular ligament reconstruction. There is no consensus as to the best method and expected outcome. This is not an operation for the uninitiated.

Preventing Monteggia Fracture-Dislocations

The best treatment of a chronic Monteggia lesion is prevention. This requires careful examination of forearm and elbow injuries to prevent missed diagnoses. Acute treatment needs to concentrate on reduction and stabilization of the forearm fracture and proximal radioulnar joint. Internal fixation is indicated for unstable, complete fractures of the ulna.

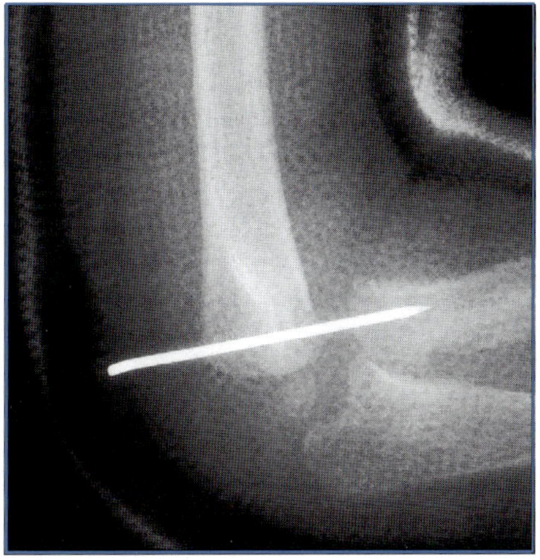

Figure 3 Reconstruction of a chronic Monteggia fracture-dislocation performed at an outside institution shows unsuccessful reduction of the radial head despite radiocapitellar pin fixation.

Case Management and Outcome Summary

After an extensive discussion with her parents regarding the risks and benefits of surgery, the patient underwent surgical reconstruction of her ulnar malunion and radial head dislocation via an extensive posterolateral approach. The radial nerve was identified, noted to be compressed by the dislocated radial head, and decompressed to the level of the posterior interosseous branch. The posterolateral capsule was incised, and the thickened, displaced annular ligament

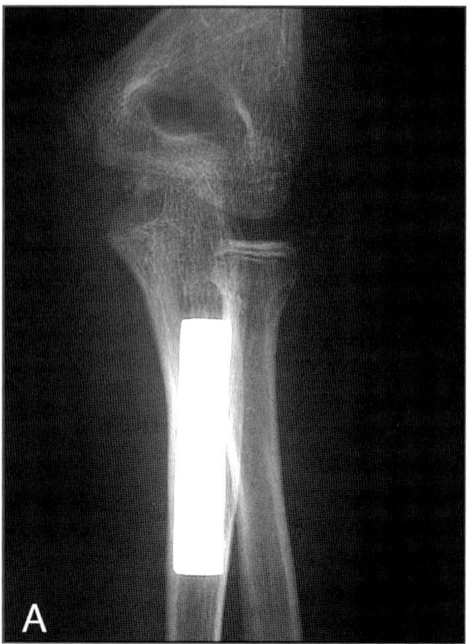

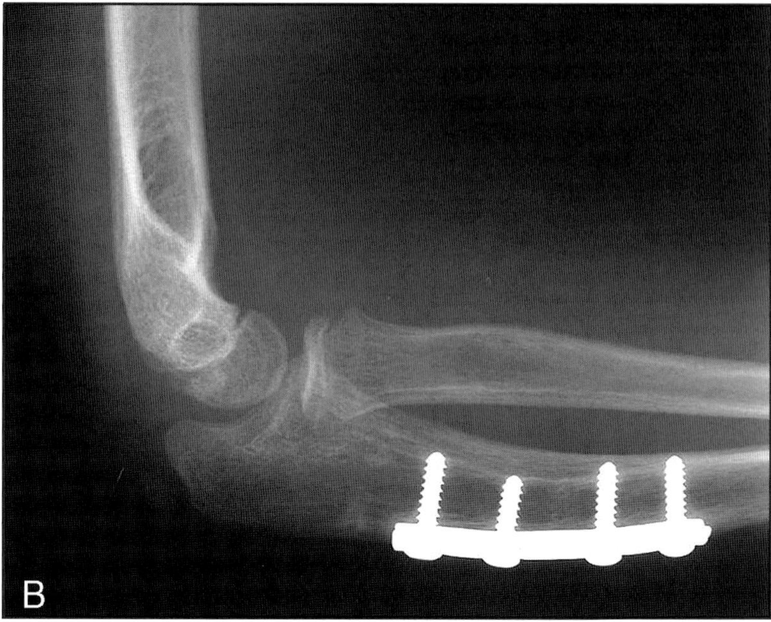

Figure 4 Example case: Postoperative AP **(A)** and lateral **(B)** radiographs 2 years after ulnar osteotomy, open reduction of the radial head, and annular ligament repair.

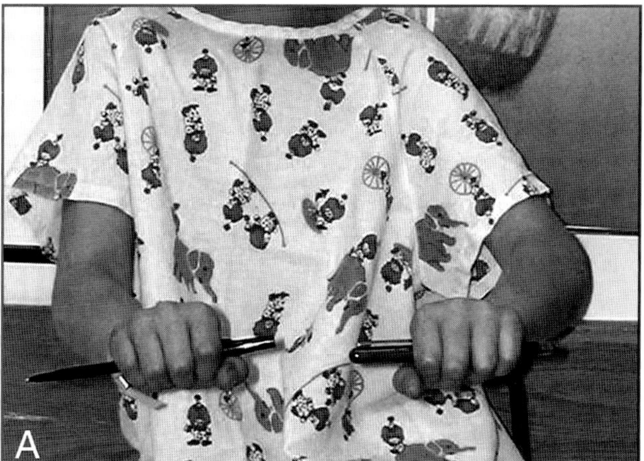

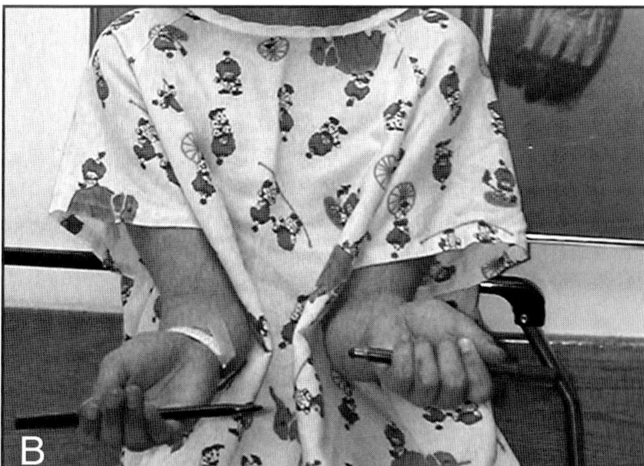

Figure 5 Example case: Postoperative pronation **(A)** and supination **(B)** of the hands of the patient whose radiographs are shown in Figures 1 and 4 at the time of planned hardware removal 2 years after reconstruction.

was extracted from the joint. The radial head was dislocated through the anterior capsule, and careful reduction into the elbow joint was performed while protecting the posterior interosseous nerve.

The proximal radioulnar and radiocapitellar joints were then débrided. It was clear that the radial head would not reduce without an ulnar osteotomy. Distal exposure of the malunited fracture site was performed. The osteotomy was performed through the healed fracture site, followed by anatomic reduction and internal fixation with a neutralization plate and screws, accentuating the ulnar bow. The radial head could easily be reduced at this stage. The annular ligament was draped over the radial neck after re-creating the normal lasso to the centrally collapsed ligament. The ligament was repaired to the ulna through the periosteum and bone. In the operating room, the patient had stable elbow flexion and extension and full forearm pronation and supination with radial head stability. The capsule and extensor supinator muscle origin was reattached.

The patient was immobilized in a bulky bivalved long arm cast for 6 weeks followed by home therapy. By 3 months after surgery, full motion and strength were restored with maintenance of anatomic reduction of her radial head. Final radiographs (Figure 4) and clinical examination (Figure 5) are noted at the time of ulnar hardware removal 2 years later.

Strategies to Minimize Common Complications

This patient was managed successfully with open joint reduction, annular ligament reconstruction, and corrective ulnar osteotomy. Fortunately, there were no perioperative complications or long-term loss of function or motion. The best initial management for this patient would have been acute recognition and surgery because at that time, the procedure and the risks would have been less serious.

References

1. Smith FM: Monteggia fractures: An analysis of 25 consecutive fresh injuries. *Surg Gynecol Obstet* 1947; 85:630-640.
2. Storen G: Traumatic dislocation of radial head as an isolated lesion in children. *Acta Chir Scand* 1956-1959;116:144-147.
3. Miles KA, Finlay DBL: Disruption of the radio-capitellar line in the normal elbow. *Injury* 1989;20: 365-367.
4. Gleeson AP, Beattie TF: Monteggia fracture-dislocation in children. *J Accid Emerg Med* 1994;11:192-194.
5. Weisman DS, Rang M, Cole WG: Tardy displacement of traumatic radial head dislocation in childhood. *J Pediatr Orthop* 1999;19:523-526.
6. Fowles JV, Sliman N, Kassah MT: The Monteggia lesion in children. *J Bone Joint Surg Am* 1983;65: 1276-1283.
7. Tait G, Sulaiman SK: Isolated dislocation of the radial head: A report of two cases. *Injury* 1988;19:125-126.
8. Best TN: Management of old unreduced Monteggia fracture dislocations of the elbow in children. *J Pediatr Orthop* 1994;14:193-199.
9. Devnani AS: Missed Monteggia fracture dislocation in children. *Injury* 1997;28:131-133.
10. Ring D, Jupiter JB, Waters PM: Monteggia fractures in children and adults. *J Am Acad Orthop Surg* 1998;6:215-224.
11. Ring D, Waters PM: Operative fixation of Monteggia fractures in children. *J Bone Joint Surg Br* 1996;78: 734-739.
12. Wise RA: Lateral dislocation of the head of radius with fracture of the ulna. *J Bone Joint Surg Am* 1941; 23:379.
13. Tompkins DG: The anterior Monteggia facture. *J Bone Joint Surg Am* 1971;53:1109-1114.
14. Morris A: Irreducible Monteggia lesion with radial nerve entrapment. *J Bone Joint Surg Am* 1974;56: 1744-1746.
15. Watson JA, Singer GC: Irreducible Monteggia fracture: Beware nerve entrapment. *Injury* 1994;25:325-327.
16. Naylor A: Monteggia fractures. *Br J Surg* 1942;29:323.
17. Stelling F, Cote R: Traumatic dislocation of head of radius in children. *JAMA* 1956;160:732-736.
18. Fahey JJ: Fractures of the elbow in children: Monteggia's fracture-dislocation. *Instr Course Lect* 1960; 17:39.
19. Austin R: Tardy palsy of the radial nerve from a Monteggia fracture. *Injury* 1926;7:202-204.
20. Hume AL: Anterior dislocation and fracture of olecranon. *J Bone Joint Surg Br* 1957;39:508-512.
21. Hurst LC, Dubrow EN: Surgical treatment of symptomatic chronic radial head dislocation: A neglected Monteggia fracture. *J Pediatr Orthop* 1983;3:227-230.
22. Kalamchi A: Monteggia fracture-dislocation in children: Late treatment in two cases. *J Bone Joint Surg Am* 1986;68:615-619.
23. Stoll TM, Willis RB, Paterson DC: Comment: Treatment of the missed Monteggia fracture in the child. *J Bone Joint Surg Br* 1992;74: 436-440.
24. Givon U, Pritsch M, Levy O, Yosepovich A, Amit Y, Horoszowski H: Monteggia and equivalent lesions: A study of 41 cases. *Clin Orthop* 1997;337:208-215.
25. Lincoln TL, Mubarak SJ: "Isolated" traumatic radial head dislocation. *J Pediatr Orthop* 1994;14:454-457.

Chapter 5

Lateral Condyle Fracture Nonunion

Kenneth J. Noonan, MD

Case Presentation

History

A right-handed 8-year-old boy who injured his left elbow after falling from overhead bars was taken to the emergency department where AP and lateral radiographs revealed a lateral condyle fracture (Figure 1). The AP view showed that the fracture line extended into the joint with lateral displacement of the fracture fragment. There was no significant displacement on the lateral view. The fracture was considered minimally displaced at that time, and the elbow was immobilized in a posterior fiberglass splint.

At follow-up 3 weeks later, the patient's pain had decreased, as had the swelling. Radiographs obtained at this time showed a slight increase in fracture displacement (Figure 2). Periosteal callus formation was noted laterally, yet no significant healing across the fracture site was observed. The boy's arm was then immobilized in a long arm cast for 1 month. Radiographs at that time revealed little healing, so his arm was immobilized for another 5 weeks, after which time progressive range of motion was started. Within 2 months, motion had returned, and the patient was able to participate in most activities. However, he reported moderate pain with lifting and pushing heavy objects.

Current Problem and Treatment

At 6 months, the patient was seen in the hand clinic where physical examination revealed an increase in his carrying angle compared with the contralateral side. His hand examination was unremarkable, and no intrinsic atrophy or increase in two-point discrimination was noted. A fluoroscopic image revealed nonunion of the lateral condyle with a "collar sign" of exuberant metaphyseal bone[1] (Figure 3). Surgery was recommended to repair the nonunion.

Discussion

Recognizing the Problem and Situations at High Risk

Lateral condyle fractures are the second most common pediatric elbow fracture and comprise 10% to 20% of all pediatric elbow fractures.[2] Fractures predominately result from a fall and an applied varus moment that leads to avulsion of

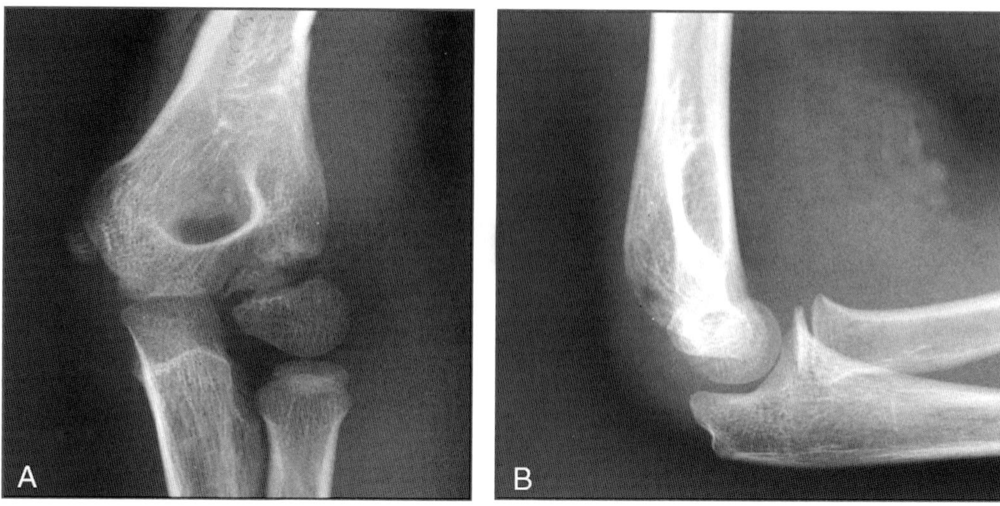

Figure 1 Example case: AP **(A)** and lateral **(B)** radiographs of the left elbow show a minimally displaced lateral condyle fracture that extends into the articular surface.

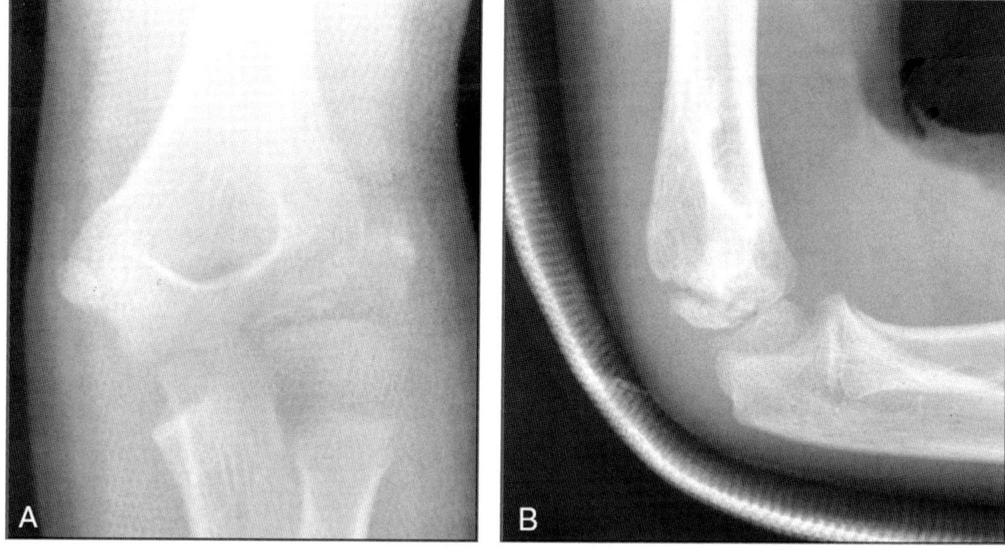

Figure 2 Example case: AP **(A)** and lateral **(B)** radiographs of the elbow 21 days after fracture. The arm had been immobilized in a posterior splint. Note the further displacement on the lateral view.

the lateral condyle by the common extensor origin. Lateral condyle fractures have been reported to occur more frequently in patients with varus malunited supracondylar fractures.[3-5]

These fractures are rare[2,6] and can be considered Salter-Harris type IV fractures as a result of an axial shear-type fracture. The more common lateral condyle fractures are the result of avulsion forces and represent a fracture plane that starts adjacent to the metaphysis and continues along the growth plate of the capitellum into the joint medial to the lateral edge of the trochlea. Complications include nonunion of

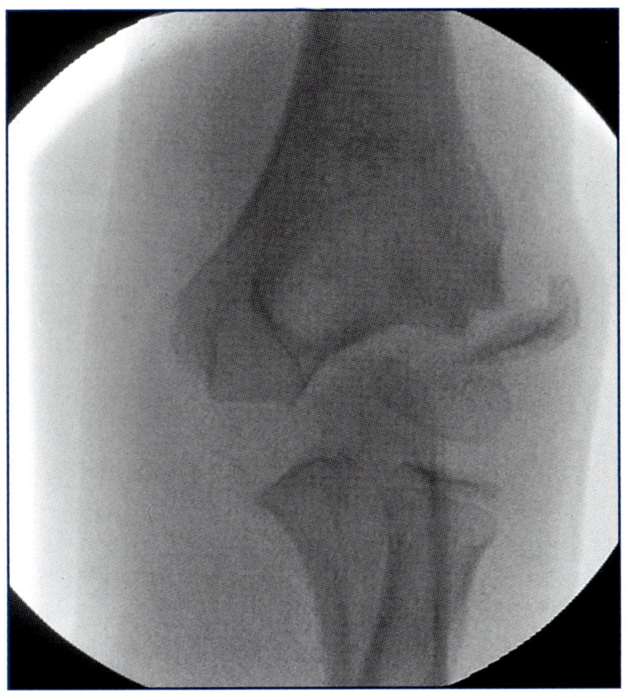

Figure 3 Example case: Fluoroscopic image obtained 6 months after the initial injury. No signs of healing are present, and further displacement confirms nonunion. The large metaphyseal fragment has a classic appearance of well-corticated bone.

the lateral condyle, osteonecrosis of the capitellum, fishtail deformity of the distal humerus, premature growth arrest of the capitellum physis, progressive lateral overgrowth and cubitus varus, and lateral prominence of the distal humerus.

Late presentation (more than 1 year) of lateral condyle fracture nonunion is a direct result of inappropriate initial treatment.[1] Compared to severe widely displaced fractures with intra-articular incongruity, minimally displaced fractures are more likely to be treated inappropriately, with resultant nonunion (13% incidence of nonunion in benign-appearing fractures).[7] Lateral condyle fractures are susceptible to progressive displacement and nonunion for several reasons. The lateral fragment is prone to further displacement because of pull of the common wrist and finger extensor origin. Furthermore, bone healing may be delayed because of poor blood supply, the relatively small amount of cortical bone available for healing, and, perhaps, poor organization of fracture hematoma from synovial fluid.[8]

It is practical to evaluate the literature regarding recent nonunions (within 1 year of fracture) separately from that regarding fractures considered long-standing. The natural history of long-standing nonunion is not known with certainty because there must certainly be individuals with unrecognized lateral condyle nonunion. Although articular incongruity is typically a predisposing factor for degenerative arthrosis, a strong relationship between nonunion and later elbow arthrosis is not evident. Other symptoms of nonunion include excessive valgus of the elbow that with time may lead to ulnar nerve palsy. Mechanical symptoms may predominate in the earlier years following a nonunion, specifically elbow instability, pain, and apprehension; functional elbow motion is usually well maintained.

Management of Lateral Condyle Fracture Nonunion

Even though the natural history of a nonunion is not firmly established, treatment of recent nonunion or "tight nonunion" is recommended because the methods to promote union are fairly reproducible.[9,10] An elbow with a well-united lateral condyle will certainly function more reliably than an elbow with an established nonunion.[10] Although case reports of healing with pulsed electromagnetic field stimulation exist,[11] surgical reconstruction is the most reliable means to correct the problem.

Flynn and associates[7] recommend repair of the recent nonunion that persists after 12 weeks. Surgical methods include isolated percutaneous screw placement across the nonunion site, if the fragment is not widely displaced.[12] Open reduction with removal of fibrous nonunion, bone grafting, and osteosynthesis with Kirschner wires (K-wires) or screws is needed for more displaced fragments. Screws are effective because they provide compression and are easy to place in the metaphyseal fragment of nonunions because of the hypertrophic bone formation.[1] This approach is used in the case presentation because use of a screw in the thin metaphyseal fragment directly after the fracture would have been difficult. In these cases pins are required.

The goal of treatment is to provide solid fusion with minimal morbidity to the elbow.[13] Care is taken to avoid associated soft-tissue damage while removing enough of the fibrous nonunion to promote bony fusion. Aggressive anatomic reduction of the nonunion should be avoided to prevent osteonecrosis.[13] Fascial lengthening of the common extensor mechanism has been described as an adjunct to decrease tension in the common extensor tendon that develops when the fragment is reduced.[14]

Lateral humeral condyle growth abnormalities consist of either growth arrest[15] of the capitellar physis or progressive varus as a result of growth stimulation.[5,9,16-19] Growth arrest is rare, but it is possible if a lateral screw is placed through the capitellum into the distal humerus. Growth stimulation and progressive varus have been documented in up to 37% of cases, with a higher incidence noted in children who are younger than age 9 years.[6]

Hasler and von Laer[20] reviewed the literature to date and detected a 16% incidence of lateral overgrowth in patients treated with open reduction and pinning with K-wires as opposed to a negligible rate of overgrowth in patients treated with screw osteosynthesis. These authors suggest that lateral overgrowth may be prevented with appropriately placed screws. They and other authors have documented prominence of the lateral condyle, which may be due to an osteoperiosteal flap and make any residual varus appear worse.[5] Even though some authors have documented high rates of lateral overgrowth, the clinical implications are slight and consist primarily of cosmetic complaints of elbow varus.

Fishtail deformities are a radiographic finding with unknown clinical significance. It has been noted that the atrophy of the center of the distal humerus may be U- or V-shaped. Theories as to the cause include perturbations of distal humeral vascularity and subsequent growth caused by trauma. Although noted at long-term follow-up, the clinical significance is negligible.

Preventing Lateral Condyle Fracture Nonunion

Treatment of lateral condyle fractures depends on the degree of displacement; nonsurgical methods are appropriate for nondisplaced fractures, but open reduction and internal fixation is needed in widely displaced fractures. Cast immobilization, percutaneous fixation, or open treatment may be effective in fractures with intermediate displacement. Closed methods are clearly preferable, if possible, to be certain that posterolateral displacement and resultant nonunion does not occur.

Jakob and associates[21] classified these fractures as nondisplaced or type 1 (1 to 2 mm of fracture diastasis) fractures. These fractures are not likely to have further displacement because the articular surface is presumed to be intact. Type 2 fractures have lateral displacement greater than 2 mm, and the joint surface is usually disrupted with the potential for further displacement. Type 3 fractures are significantly displaced, with displacement of the radiocapitellar joint. Both this classification system and that of Badelon and associates[16] have identified fractures that are minimally displaced and at low risk for further displacement and nonunion.

I recommend that fracture displacement be quantified on AP, lateral, and oblique radiographs, and that the maximum displacement or lateral translation[22] on any of the three views be used to guide treatment. Flynn and associates[7] reported that fractures with displacement greater than or equal to 3 mm would likely lead to nonunion. Finnbogason and associates[23] reviewed 112 fractures with less than 2 mm of displacement and then studied the fracture plane and its relationship to further displacement. Stable fractures did not extend to the joint and had no further displacement. Uncertain fractures extended into the joint, but the fracture surfaces tended to converge; late displacement occurred in 17% of these fractures. Unstable fractures displaced 42% of the time and were considered unstable because the fracture surfaces had parallel displacement of 2 mm into the joint. Despite the excellent work above, radiographic interpretation is subjective, and the potential for late displacement exists in 10% of fractures that are considered minimally displaced on radiographs.[7,16,24] Therefore, some investigators have attempted to use other methods to assess the stability of minimally displaced fractures.

Stress radiographs may be of some use in predicting future displacement but require an extremely compliant child or heavy sedation. Arthrography is sometimes used as an adjunct to determine the integrity of the articular surface prior to treatment or as a method to assess reduction from closed reduction.[25] Marzo and associates[22] reported that arthrography is a useful and accurate test for predicting further displacement of the

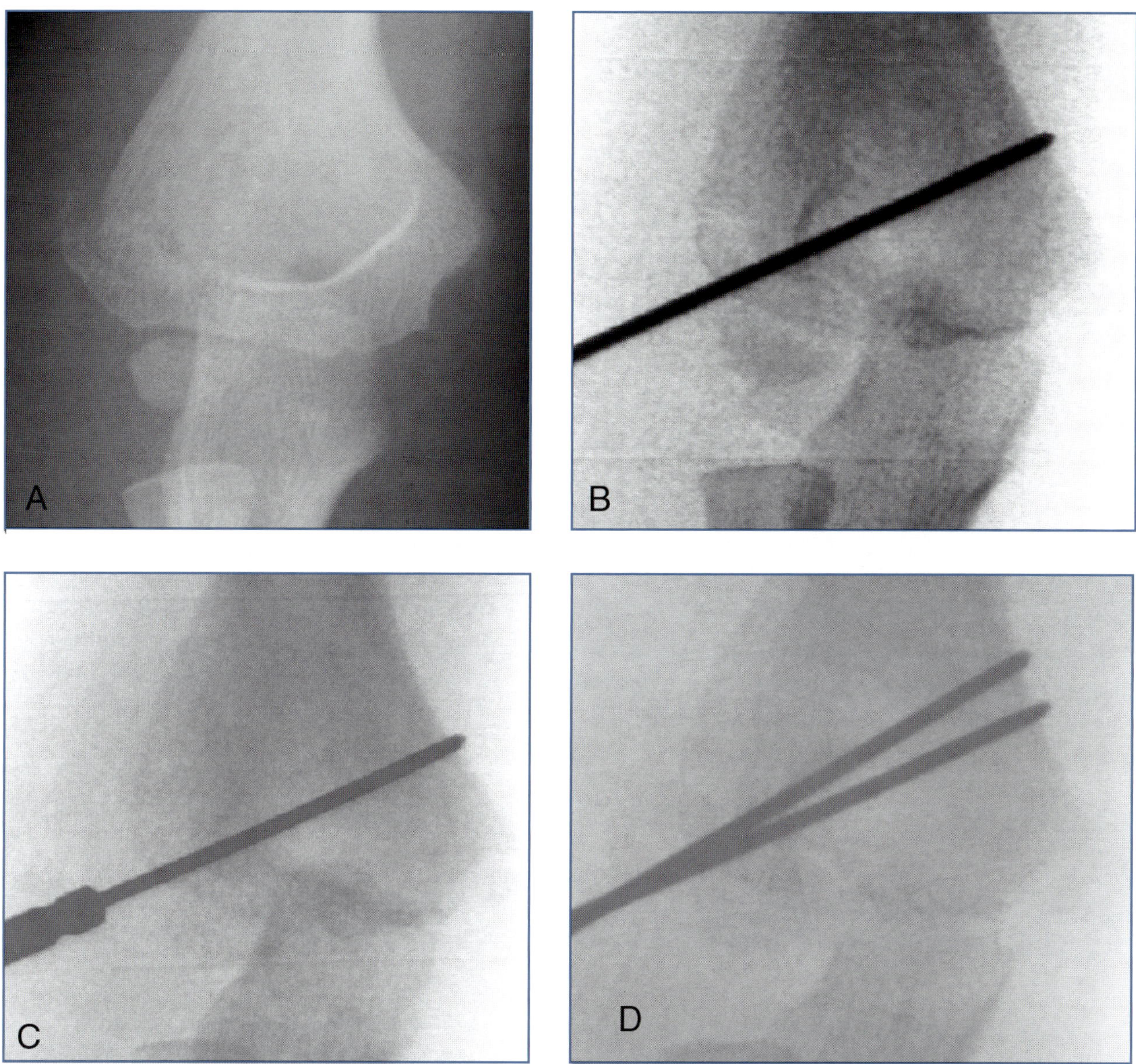

Figure 4 A, Percutaneous reduction and compression of a lateral condyle fracture. **B,** Manual reduction and pinning is performed. **C,** A reversed 4.5-mm cannulated drill bit is used to further compress the fracture. **D,** A second pin is introduced to maintain reduction.

fracture surface. The sensitivity of detecting intra-articular extension was 92%; however, the potential for false-negative results exists if hematoma formation in the fracture site blocks dye migration into the fracture line. I believe that arthrography is most useful as an adjunct to assessing fracture reduction after closed reduction and percutaneous pinning. If articular integrity is the key to fracture stability, MRI may be a useful method to predict further displacement. Two recent studies have proved that if the fracture line does not extend into the joint, no further displacement occurs.[26,27] This technology is appealing, yet it is possi-

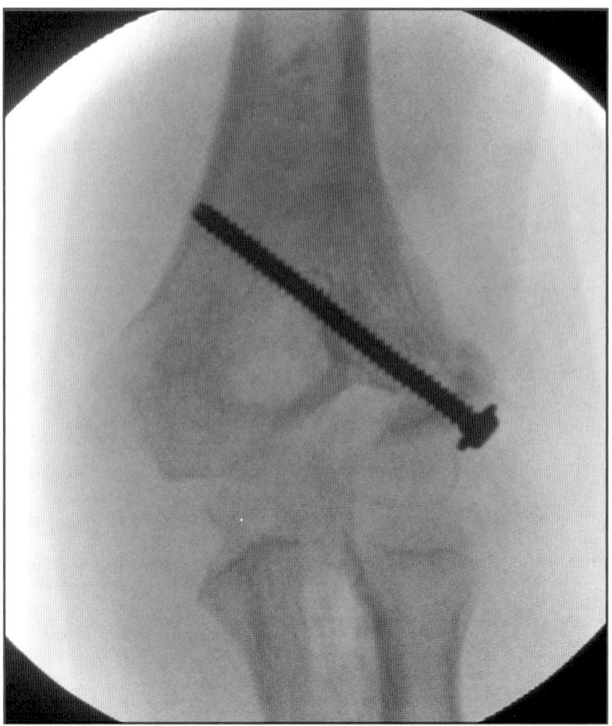

Figure 5 Example case: Intraoperative fluoroscopic image demonstrates partial reduction of the lateral condyle with a cannulated screw across the metaphyseal fragment. Cancellous bone graft was taken from the proximal ulna and placed into the nonunion site.

ble to argue that the benefit of MRI does not outweigh the cost and potential need for sedation.

Long arm cast immobilization is recommended in all fractures that have less than 2 mm of displacement on all three radiographic views. Although MRI may document the integrity of the joint surface, I recommend close radiographic follow-up to detect further displacement. Patients are scheduled to return for follow-up 5 days after the fracture occurred for three views of the distal humerus with the arm out of the cast. Lacking displacement, treatment in a long arm cast is continued, and the child returns for repeat radiographs with the arm out of the cast at 14 days. Cast immobilization and radiographs with the arm out of the cast are continued at 2- to 3-week intervals for up to 12 weeks until the fracture heals or further displacement occurs. Flynn and associates[7] reported that an extended period of immobilization (8 to 12 weeks) may be required in up to one third of fractures to ensure complete healing of the thin metaphyseal fragment, which occurs primarily by endosteal healing. The above treatment protocol is effective in 98% of patients with fresh lateral condyle fractures that are truly displaced less than 2 mm on all three radiographic views.[28] Surgical fixation should be considered in fractures that displace more than 2 mm or fail to heal in appropriate time.

Treatment options for fractures with more than 2 mm of initial displacement or minimally displaced fractures that gradually displace despite closed treatment consist of either closed or open reduction and stabilization. Osteosynthesis may be performed with K-wires or screw fixation. Closed reduction and percutaneous fixation is useful for fresh displaced fractures or for older fractures that have progressive displacement in a cast.[9,29,30] Fluoroscopic reduction is performed under anesthesia with the elbow flexed and the hand supinated. Manual reduction may be aided with a percutaneously placed K-wire as a joystick. The fragment may be compressed by sliding a reversed cannulated drill bit over the first K-wire while a second divergent K-wire is introduced (Figure 4). Alternatively, compression may be obtained with a percutaneously placed screw. Reduction can then be assessed with multiple fluoroscopic images or with an arthrogram. Open reduction and internal fixation can be considered should displacement of the joint be deemed unacceptable after closed reduction and stabilization. Newer methods of closed treatment and percutaneous fixation are in contradistinction to previous recommendations of open reduction and fixation for all fractures that are displaced more than 2 to 3 mm.[1,7,9,16,24] Bhandari and associates[31] recently conducted an evidence-based analysis of closed reduction and percutaneous pinning and arthrogram versus open reduction and internal fixation. Based on this analysis they could not support either as the preferred method.

Open reduction and internal fixation is indicated for all completely displaced fractures or those in which closed reduction failed based on fluoroscopic images or arthrograms. These procedures can be challenging, and the surgeon will need an assistant to either maintain reduction or place K-wires for ultimate fixation. A Kocher approach is developed between the triceps and brachioradialis. Imprudent dissection posterior to the lateral condyle will predispose for osteonecrosis of

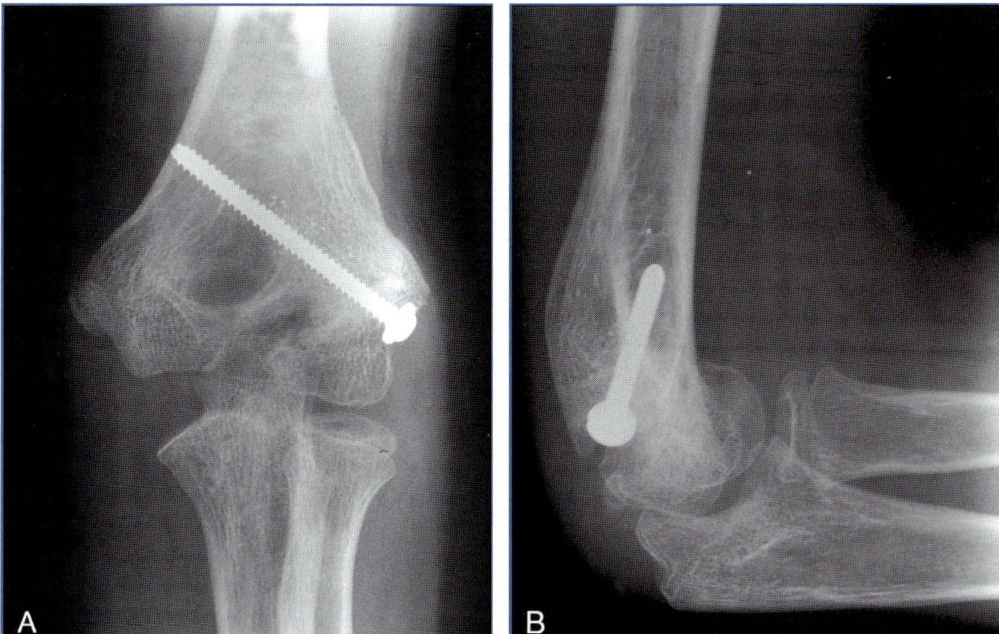

Figure 6 Example case: AP **(A)** and lateral **(B)** radiographs obtained 1 year after surgical repair of the nonunion. Note the complete bone bridging from the metaphysis to the fragment on the AP view.

the capitellum. The approach can be extended into the anterior joint capsule, allowing assessment of joint congruity. The fragment is stabilized with two or three smooth wires placed across the metaphyseal fragment into the proximal humerus. Skeletal fixation is supplemented with cast immobilization until the fracture appears fully healed on radiographs.

Thomas and associates[5] suggested that 3 weeks of K-wire fixation and casting are sufficient to ensure healing prior to gradual therapy. However, most authors recommend maintaining the pins until radiographic healing is evident, which is usually by 6 weeks.[29] Other authors have reported good results with a screw placed across the metaphyseal portion of the lateral condylar fragment.[20,32,33] This method is reasonable provided that the metaphyseal fragment is large enough to support the screw[5] and prevent growth arrest of the physis of the capitellum.

Case Management and Outcome Summary

A lateral Kocher approach was used, and great care was taken to avoid significant posterior stripping while the fibrocartilaginous material was removed from the nonunion site of the metaphysis. No attempt was made to remove all of the nonunion material down to the articular surface, and complete reduction of the fragment was not planned. Cancellous bone graft was obtained through a separate incision over the proximal ulna and placed into the metaphyseal region. A 4.0-mm cortical screw was lagged across the nonunion site, providing compression (Figure 5).

The patient's arm was immobilized in a long arm cast for 6 weeks, at which time radiographs revealed early healing, and he was started on range-of-motion exercises. After 1 year, the patient had a 15° extension contracture with full flexion, and radiographs confirmed healing of the nonunion at the metaphysis (Figure 6). After 2 years, the patient had a 5° lack of terminal extension and had returned to all activities without pain, apprehension, or instability (Figure 7).

Strategies to Minimize Common Complications

This case is illustrative of issues encountered in management that resulted in fracture nonunion. First, the

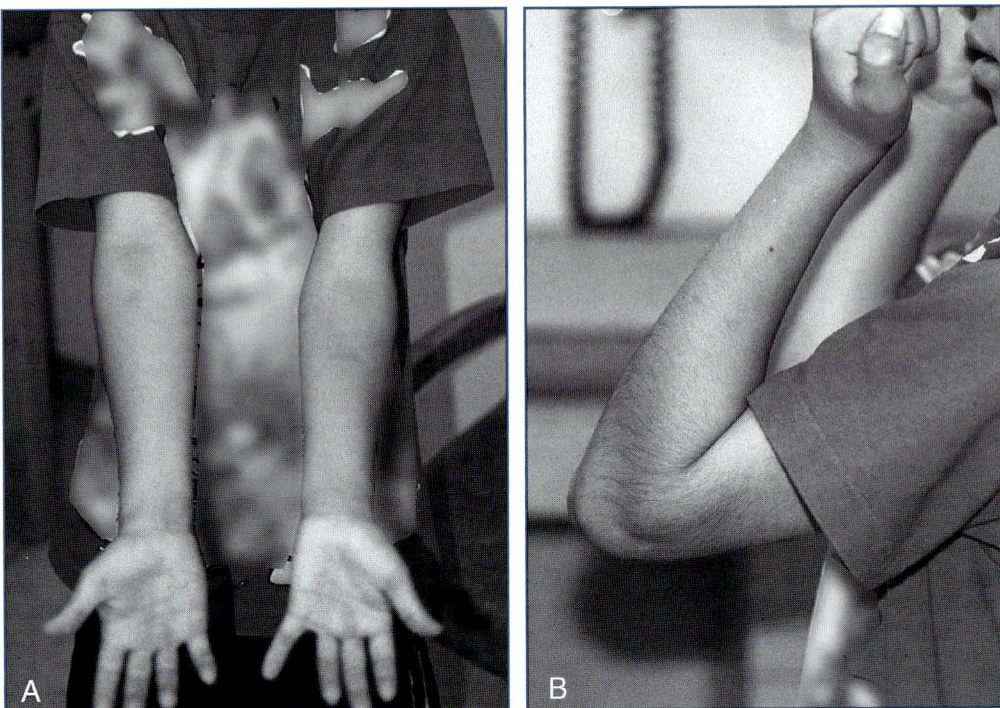

Figure 7 Example case: AP **(A)** and lateral **(B)** clinical photographs obtained at 2-year follow-up demonstrate no significant difference in carrying angle and near full extension and full elbow flexion.

initial radiographs were not complete (no oblique view) or assessed properly (more than 2 mm of lateral displacement). Second, this fracture should be considered at high risk for repeat displacement as a result of the parallel nature of the intra-articular fracture surfaces.[5,23] The patient was immobilized in a splint with extended follow-up. Further displacement was noted at 3 weeks and required surgical fixation at that point.

References

1. Flynn JC, Richards JF Jr: Nonunion of minimally displaced fractures of the lateral condyle of humerus in children. *J Bone Joint Surg Am* 1971;53:1096-1101.
2. Mirsky EC, Karas EH, Weiner LS: Lateral condyle fractures in children: Evaluation of classification and treatment. *J Orthop Trauma* 1997;11:117-120.
3. Davids JR, Maguire MF, Mubarak SJ, Wenger DR: Lateral condylar fracture of the humerus following posttraumatic cubitus varus. *J Pediatr Orthop* 1994;14:466-470.
4. Takahara M, Sasaki I, Kimura T, Kato H, Minami A, Ogino T: Second fracture of the distal humerus after varus malunion of a supracondylar fracture in children. *J Bone Joint Surg Br* 1998;80:791-796.
5. Thomas DP, Howard AW, Cole WG, Hedden DM: Three weeks of Kirschner wire fixation for displaced lateral condylar fractures of the humerus in children. *J Pediatr Orthop* 2001;21:565-569.
6. Skak SV, Olsen SD, Smaabrekke A: Deformity after fracture of the lateral humeral condyle in children. *J Pediatr Orthop* 2001;10:142-152.
7. Flynn JC, Richards JF Jr, Saltzmann RI: Prevention and treatment of non-union of slightly displaced fractures of the lateral humeral condyle in children: An end-result study. *J Bone Joint Surg Am* 1975;57:1087-1092.
8. Hardacre JA, Nahigian SH, Froimson AI, et al: Fractures of the lateral condyle of the humerus in children. *J Bone Joint Surg Am* 1971;53:1083-1095.
9. Foster DE, Sullivan JA, Gross RH: Lateral humeral condylar fractures in children. *J Pediatr Orthop* 1985;5:16-22.

10. DeBoeck H: Surgery for nonunion of the lateral humeral condyle in children: Six cases followed for 1-9 years. *Acta Orthop Scand* 1995;66: 401-402.
11. Sankar SD, Bassett CA: Healing of nonunion of a fractured lateral condyle of the humerus by pulsing electromagnetic induction. *Contemp Orthop* 1991;22:47-51.
12. Morris S, McKenna J, Cassidy N, Stephens M: A new technique for treatment of a non-union of a lateral humeral condyle. *Injury* 2000;31: 557-559.
13. Wattenbarger JM, Gerardi J, Johnston CE: Late open reduction internal fixation of lateral condyle fractures. *J Pediatr Orthop* 2002;22: 394-398.
14. Gauer SC, Varma AN, Swarup A: A new surgical technique for old ununited lateral condyle fractures of the humerus in children. *J Trauma* 1993;34:68-69.
15. Rutherford A: Fractures of the lateral humeral condyle in children. *J Bone Joint Surg Am* 1985;67: 851-856.
16. Badelon O, Bensahel H, Mazda K, Vie P: Lateral humeral condylar fractures in children: A report of 47 cases. *J Pediatr Orthop* 1998;8: 31-34.
17. Fahey JJ: Fractures of the elbow in children. *Instr Course Lect* 1960;17: 13-16.
18. So YC, Fang D, Leong JCY, Bong SC: Varus deformity following lateral humeral condylar fractures in children. *J Pediatr Orthop* 1985;5: 569-572.
19. Wilkins KE: Residuals of elbow trauma in children. *Orthop Clin North Am* 1990;21:291-314.
20. Hasler CC, von Laer L: Prevention of growth disturbances after fractures of the lateral humeral condyle in children. *J Pediatr Orthop* 2001; 10:123-130.
21. Jakob R, Fowles JV, Rang M, Kassab MT: Observations concerning fractures in the lateral condyles in children. *J Bone Joint Surg Br* 1975;57:430-436.
22. Marzo JM, d'Amato C, Strong M, Gillespie R: Usefulness and accuracy of arthrography in management of lateral humeral condyle fractures in children. *J Pediatr Orthop* 1990; 10:317-321.
23. Finnbogason T, Karlsson G, Lindberg L, Mortensson W: Nondisplaced and minimally displaced fractures of the lateral humeral condyle in children: A prospective radiographic investigation of fracture stability. *J Pediatr Orthop* 1995;15:422-425.
24. Flynn JC: Nonunion of slightly displaced fractures of the lateral humeral condyle in children: An update. *J Pediatr Orthop* 1989;9: 691-696.
25. Yates C, Sullivan JA: Arthrographic diagnosis of elbow injuries in children. *J Pediatr Orthop* 1987; 7:54-60.
26. Horn BD, Herman MJ, Crisci K, Pizzutillo PD, MacEwen GD: Fractures of the lateral humeral condyle: Role of the cartilage hinge in fracture stability. *J Pediatr Orthop* 2002;22:8-11.
27. Kamegaya M, Shinohara Y, Kurokawa M, Ogata S: Assessment of stability in children's minimally displaced lateral humeral condyle fracture by magnetic resonance imaging. *J Pediatr Orthop* 1999;19: 570-572.
28. Bast SC, Hoffer MM, Aval S: Nonoperative treatment for minimally and nondisplaced lateral humeral condyle fractures in children. *J Pediatr Orthop* 1998;18:448-450.
29. Cardona JI, Riddle E, Kumar SJ: Displaced fractures of the lateral humeral condyle: Criteria for implant removal. *J Pediatr Orthop* 2002;22:194-197.
30. Mintzer CM, Waters PM, Brown DJ, Kasser JR: Percutaneous pinning in the treatment of displaced lateral condyle fractures. *J Pediatr Orthop* 1994;14:462-465.
31. Bhandari M, Tornetta P, Swiontkowski M: Displaced lateral condyle fractures of the distal humerus. *J Pediatr Trauma* 2003;17:306-308.
32. Conner AN, Smith MG: Displaced fractures of the lateral humeral condyle in children. *J Bone Joint Surg Br* 1970;52:460-464.
33. Sharma JC, Arora A, Mathur NC, Gupta SP, Biyani A, Mathur R: Lateral condylar fractures of the humerus in children: Fixation with partially threaded 4.0-mm AO cancellous screws. *J Trauma* 1995;39: 1129-1133.

Chapter 6

Irreducible Radial Neck Fractures

Charles T. Price, MD

Case Presentation

History

A 10-year, 10-month-old boy sustained a displaced radial neck fracture in a fall from a bicycle (Figure 1). Closed reduction under general anesthesia was attempted using several of the methods discussed in the next section. These were unsuccessful. Open reduction with internal fixation using miniscrew fixation was performed through a lateral approach. Reduction was incomplete following internal fixation but was accepted (Figure 2). The fracture united uneventfully, and the screws were removed 12 weeks after the initial injury.

Current Problem and Treatment

Ten months after the initial injury, the patient presented for a second opinion because of clicking in his elbow. Radiographs demonstrated a united radial neck fracture with persistent translation (Figure 3). Loss of 50° of pronation was also noted but did not interfere with daily function or sporting activities. (Figure 4). He was otherwise asymptomatic.

Discussion

Recognizing the Problem and Situations at High Risk

Radial neck fractures are most common in children aged 9 to 12 years, but these fractures may occur at any age. The most common mechanism of injury is a valgus stress with compression of the radial neck. Associated fractures occur in approximately 50% of patients, but these fractures are managed independently in order to restore alignment and stability.

Management of Radial Neck Fractures

The radial neck fracture itself may be troublesome to reduce, regardless of associated injuries. Complete displacement can occur, as described in the case presentation. Angulation greater than 30° requires reduction except in very young children, when up to 45° of angulation may be accepted. However, translation may limit motion more than angulation as a result of the CAM effect

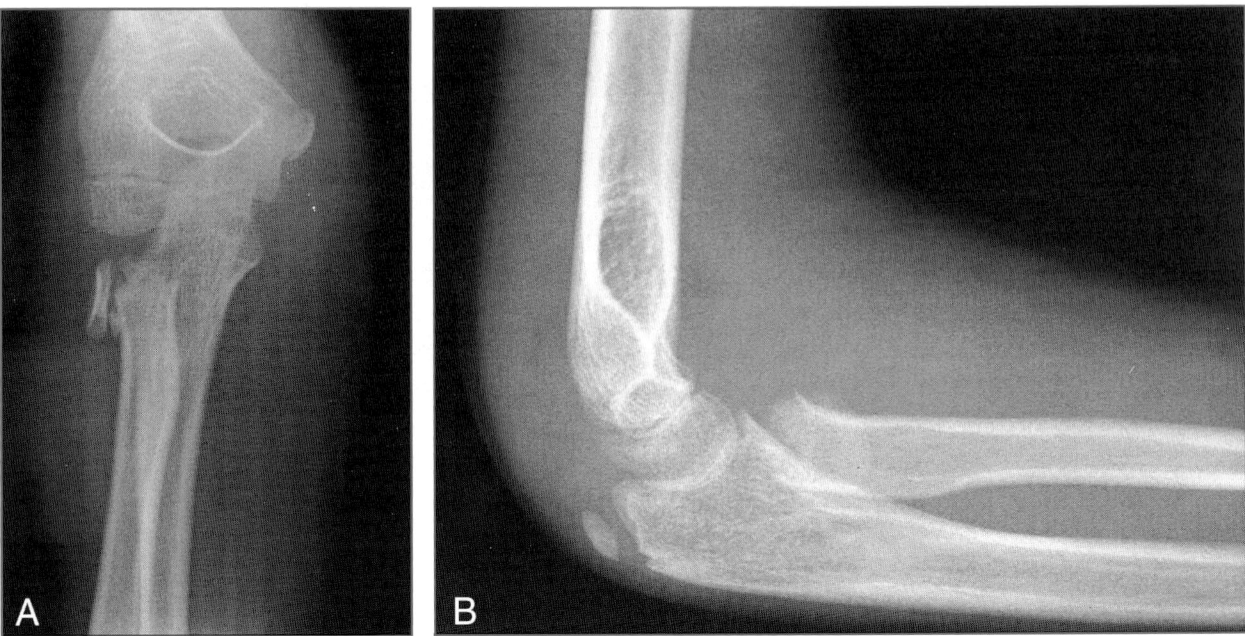

Figure 1 Example case: AP **(A)** and lateral **(B)** radiographs of the elbow of a 10-year, 10-month-old boy who sustained a completely displaced isolated fracture of the radial neck after falling from his bicycle.

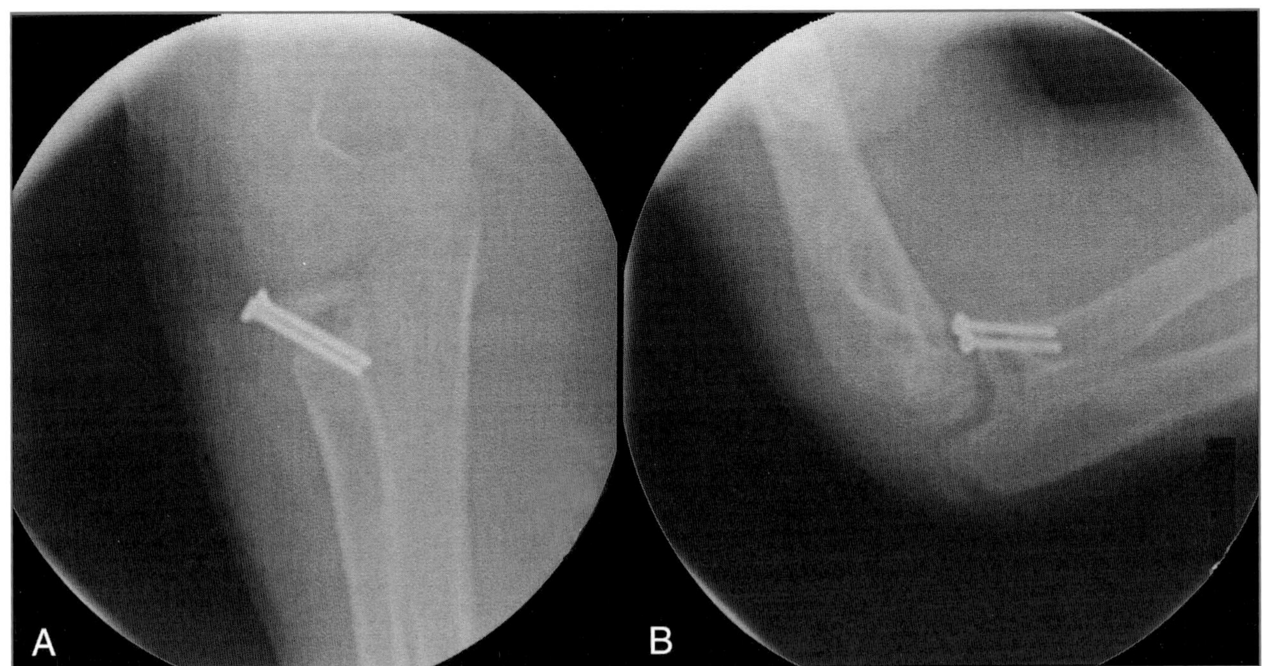

Figure 2 Example case: AP **(A)** and lateral **(B)** radiographs following open reduction and internal fixation with minifragment screws. Open reduction was necessary following several attempts at closed reduction using a variety of methods. Note that anterior translation of the fracture is still present.

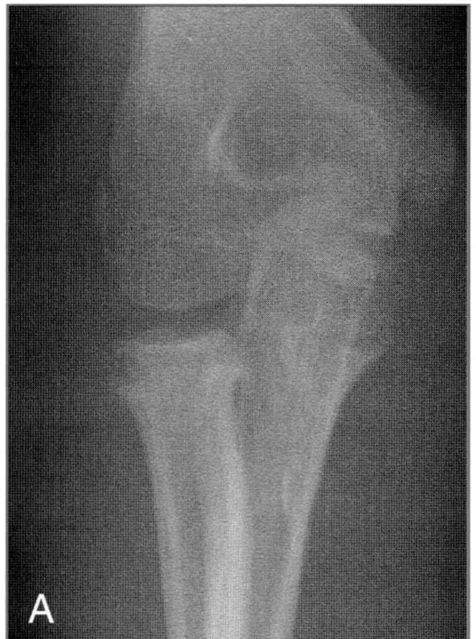

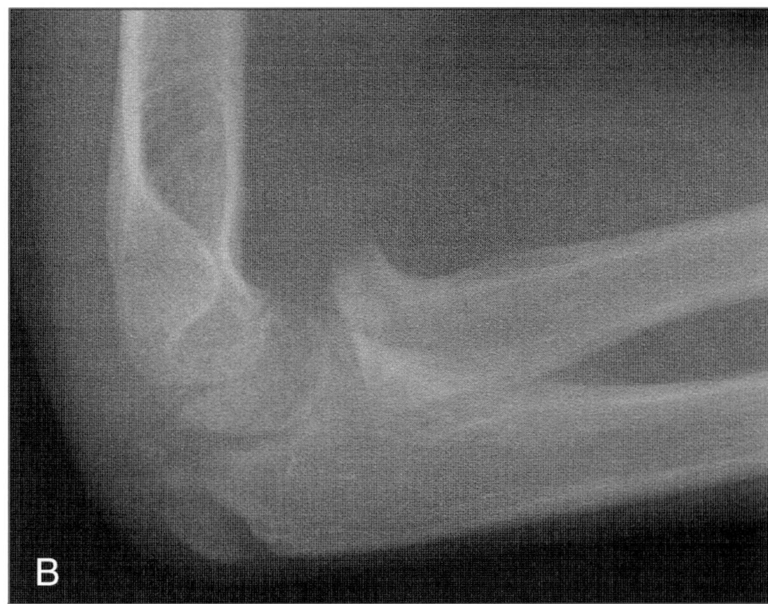

Figure 3 Example case: AP **(A)** and lateral **(B)** radiographs obtained 10 months after the initial injury demonstrate satisfactory union with persistent anterior translation of the radial head.

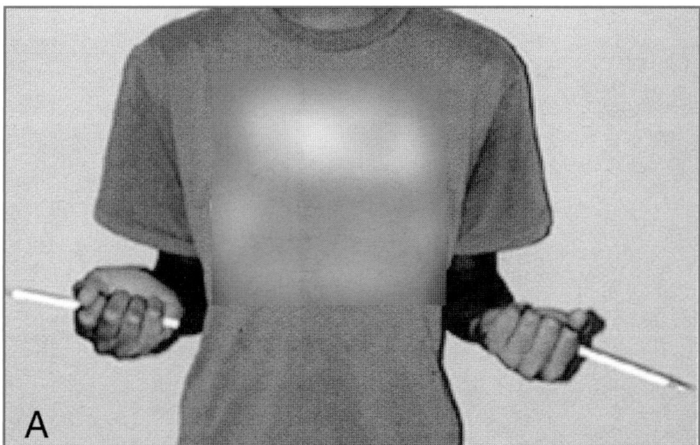

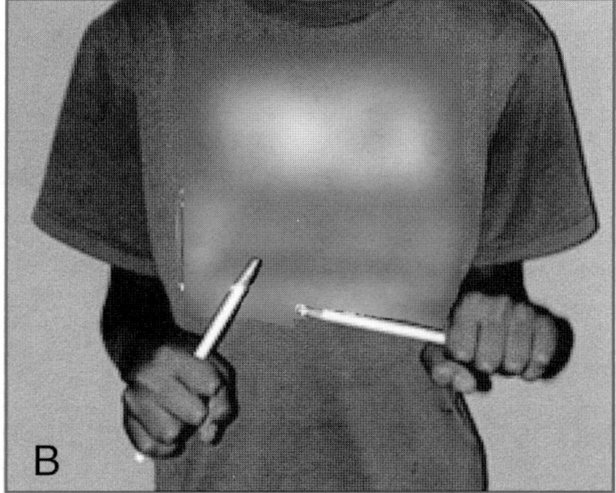

Figure 4 Example case: **A** and **B,** Clinical photographs 10 months after the initial injury. The patient reports asymptomatic "clicking" in his elbow. Note loss of forearm pronation. Loss of motion may be due to the severity of the initial trauma, the age of the patient, open reduction, incomplete reduction, or a combination thereof.

of radial neck rotation in the annular ligament. Angulation may remodel, but translation of more than 3 mm has been associated with poor results due to restriction of forearm rotation. Poor results have also been noted when the initial injury is more severe, in children older than age 10 years, when treatment is delayed, and following open reduction. For these reasons, early closed management is preferred; although it should be noted that open reduction is more likely when the initial injury is severe.[1-4]

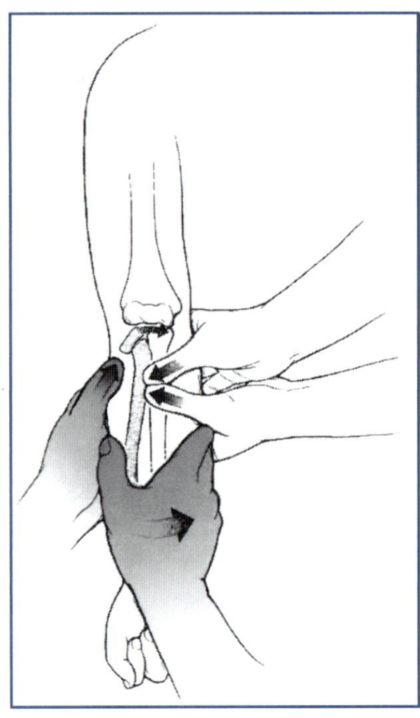

Figure 5 A recently proposed reduction technique uses laterally directed force on the radial shaft while the elbow is stressed into varus. The radial head is positioned radiographically in the plane of maximum angular displacement, and pressure is applied to the proximal fragment. (Reproduced with permission from Neher CG, Torch MA: New reduction technique for severely displaced pediatric radial neck fractures. *J Pediatr Orthop* 2003;23:626-628.)

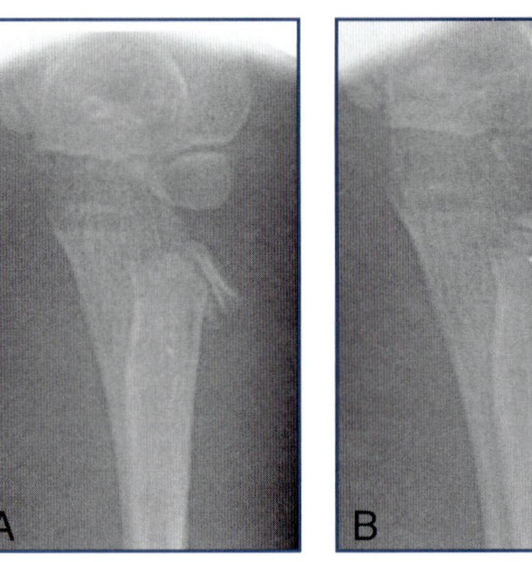

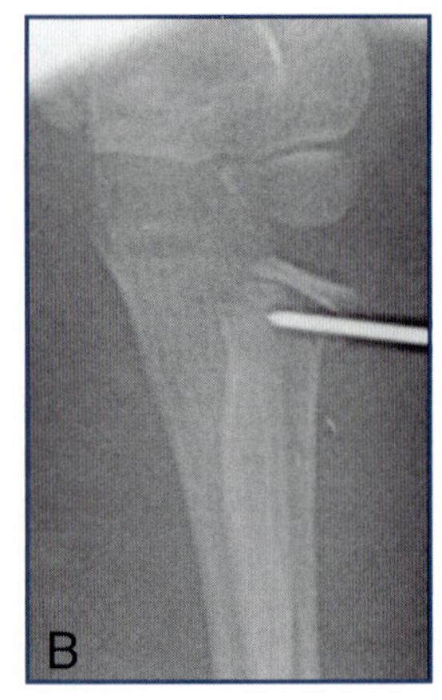

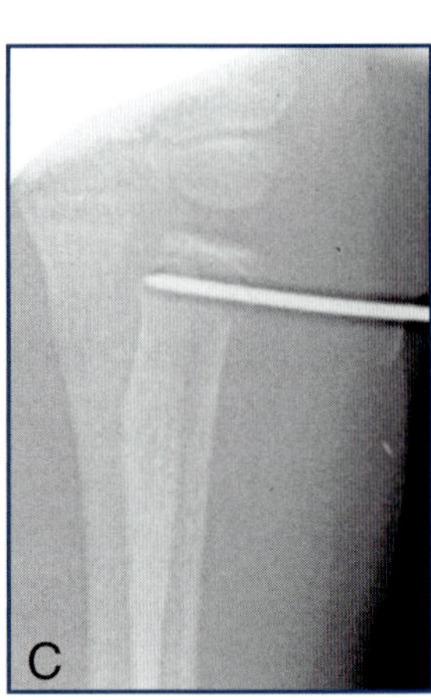

Figure 6 Fluoroscopic images during reduction of a radial neck fracture using a percutaneous pin technique. The fracture was stable following reduction and healed uneventfully in a long arm cast.

Preventing Irreducible Radial Neck Fractures

Standard closed reduction maneuvers consist of distraction with varus stress on the elbow followed by positioning of the radius to apply pressure over the radial head, forcing it back into position. This maneuver is often successful; when it fails, several other methods are available to attempt reduction. One method is to firmly apply an Esmarch bandage to the forearm to produce compression with elongation due to uniform pressure on the soft tissues. Recently, a method of applying pressure to the radial shaft has

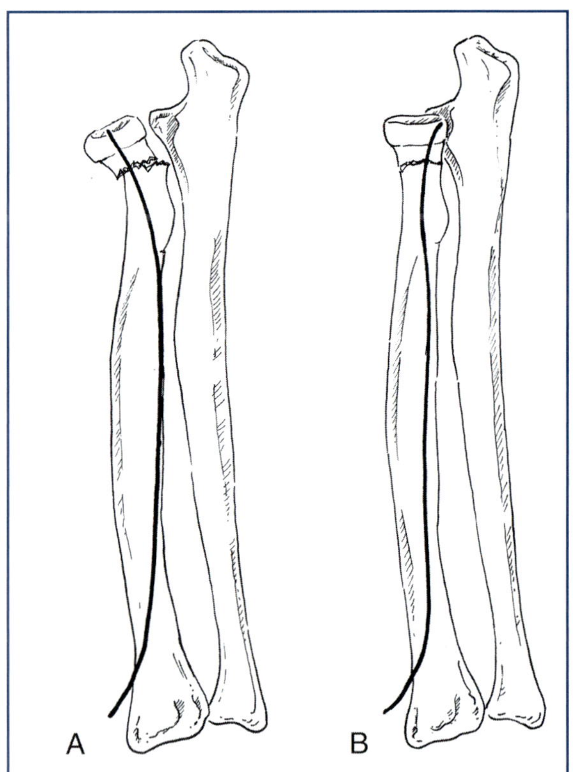

Figure 7 The Metaizeau technique for reduction and pinning of displaced radial neck fractures by closed percutaneous pinning. **A,** The flexible nail is inserted into the distal radius, passed though the intramedullary canal into the radial head. **B,** The nail is then rotated to reduce the fracture.

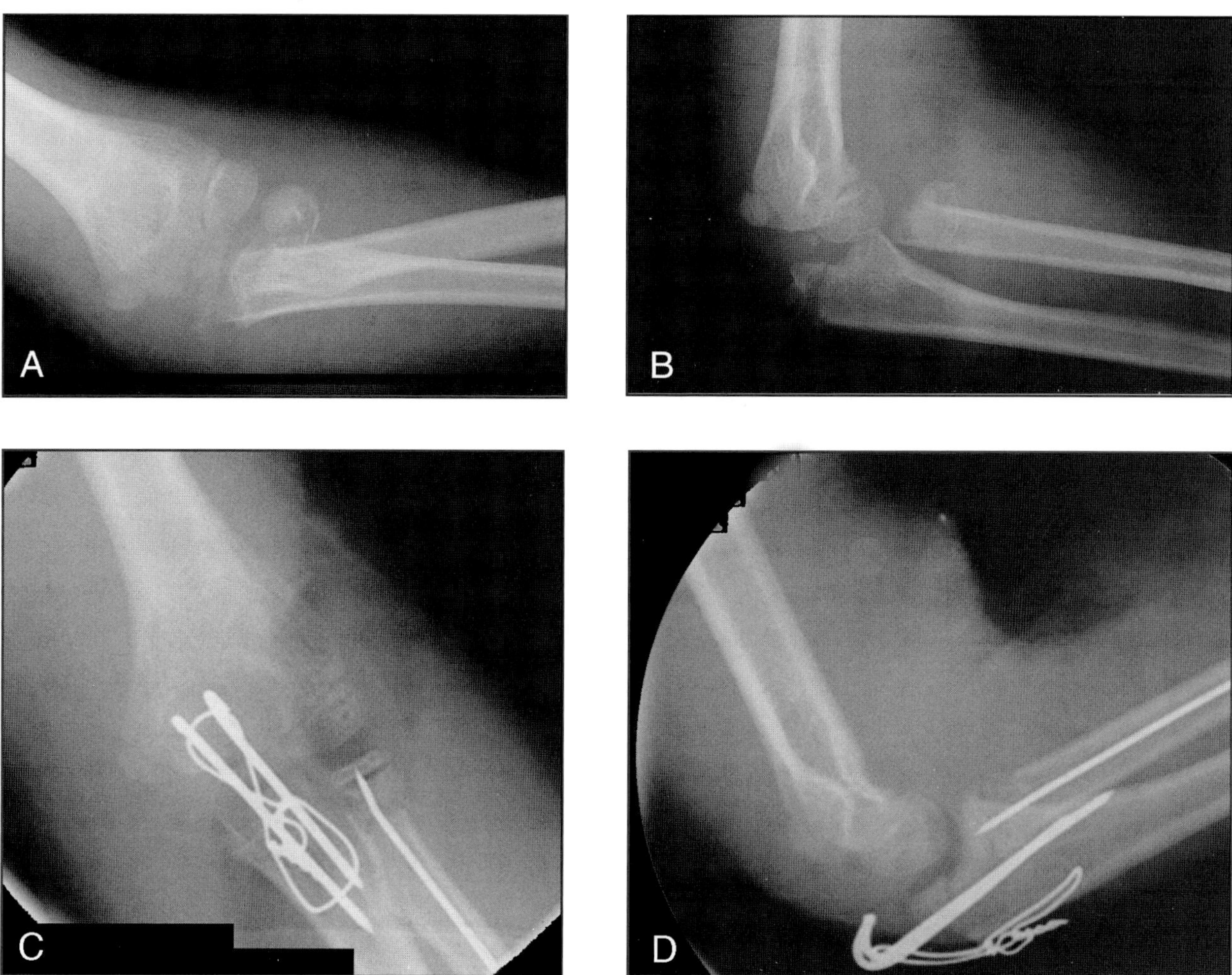

Figure 8 AP **(A)** and lateral **(B)** radiographs of an elbow fracture-dislocation. Note the severe displacement of the radial neck combined with an olecranon fracture. AP **(C)** and lateral **(D)** radiographs following open reduction and internal fixation. Note the stable fixation of the olecranon fracture with intramedullary pinning of the radial neck fracture.

been described[5] (Figure 5). If this method fails, a percutaneous incision may be considered to allow insertion of a small elevator over the radial shaft to help pull the shaft laterally while the radial head is pushed medially. At times a percutaneous pin can be inserted to manipulate the proximal fragment into an acceptable position (Figure 6).

When attempts at closed reduction have failed, the Metaizeau technique of inserting a contoured flexible nail from the distal radius may be considered.[6-8] This nail can penetrate the metaphysis of the proximal fragment when displacement is less than 100%. Then rotating the wire reduces the radial head. This technique also stabilizes the radial neck fracture during healing (Figure 7).

Open reduction is required when closed reduction has failed or when the fracture is intra-articular and involves more than one third of the joint surface. Fixation may be achieved with small Kirschner wires that are removed after 3 to 4 weeks to begin early motion. Alternatively, small screws can be used to begin early motion without early removal of implants. Another method for fixation is the Metaizeau technique even when open reduction is necessary (Figure 8). Cast immobilization for 3 weeks is advisable in most cases because stable fixation is difficult, regardless of technique.

Case Management and Outcome Summary

Persistent translation is a likely cause of the patient's complaint of clicking and may have contributed to the loss of pronation. However, his elbow motion was within acceptable limits for normal daily activities.[9] For this reason, his outcome was accepted rather than resorting to further surgery.

Strategies to Minimize Common Complications

Closed reduction or percutaneous reduction of radial neck fractures should be attempted for most fractures when angulation is greater than 30° and translation is more than 3 mm. Parents should be advised that loss of forearm rotation may result even when these fractures are reduced anatomically by closed means. However, some fractures defy closed methods and require open reduction with internal fixation. In these more severe fractures, the risk of loss of motion is increased, regardless of anatomic reduction.

Acknowledgment

I would like to thank Mark Birnbaum, MD and Jonathan Phillips, MD, of Orlando, Florida, for allowing publication of the cases used in Figures 6 and 8.

References

1. Tibone JE, Stoltz M: Fractures of the radial head and neck in children. *J Bone Joint Surg Am* 1981;63: 100-106.
2. Evans MC, Graham HK: Radial neck fractures in children: A management algorithm. *J Pediatr Orthop* 1999;8:93-99.
3. Fowles JV, Kassab MT: Observations regarding radial neck fractures in children. *J Pediatr Orthop* 1986; 6:51-57.
4. Steinberg EL, Golomb D, Salama R, Weintroub S: Radial head and neck fractures in children. *J Pediatr Orthop* 1988;8:35-40.
5. Neher CG, Torch MA: New reduction technique for severely displaced pediatric radial neck fractures. *J Pediatr Orthop* 2003;23:626-628.
6. Metaizeau JP, Lascombes P, Lemelle JL, Finlayson D, Prevot J: Reduction and fixation of displaced radial neck fractures by closed intramedullary pinning. *J Pediatr Orthop* 1993;13:355-360.
7. Gonzalez-Herranz P, Alvarez-Romera A, Burgos J, Rapariz JM, Hevia E: Displaced radial neck fractures in children treated by closed intramedullary pinning (Metaizeau technique). *J Pediatr Orthop* 1997; 17:325-331.
8. Stiefel D, Meuli M, Altermatt S: Fractures of the neck of the radius in children. *J Bone Joint Surg Br* 2001;83:536-541.
9. Morrey BF, Askew LJ, Chao EY: A biomechanical study of normal functional elbow motion. *J Bone Joint Surg Am* 1981;63:872-877.

Chapter 7

Supracondylar Humerus Fracture With Malunion

John M. Flynn, MD

Case Presentation

History

A 6-year-old girl who fell from playground equipment onto an outstretched hand sustained a type III supracondylar fracture of her right humerus (Figure 1). She was initially taken to a nearby hospital where a closed reduction and percutaneous pinning was performed. Intraoperative images after pinning were available (Figure 2). Her postoperative recovery was uneventful, and she returned to the original surgeon's office for radiographs in her cast 1 week later. These radiographs showed loss of reduction (Figure 3).

Current Problem and Treatment

The family presented for a second opinion to determine whether further surgery would be needed.

Discussion

Recognizing the Problem and Situations at High Risk

This case presentation described loss of reduction of a supracondylar humeral fracture, followed by revision of fixation to avoid malunion. Malunion of a pediatric supracondylar humeral fracture is much less common in the current era of closed reduction and pinning than it was when closed reduction and casting or olecranon traction and casting were used. Although many consider it primarily a cosmetic problem, malunion (cubitus varus) after supracondylar humeral fractures creates an unsatisfactory outcome and is a source of medical malpractice claims.

The most common malunion of a pediatric supracondylar humeral fracture is extension and cubitus varus (Figure 4). This deformity does not remodel to any satisfying extent, although some loss of elbow flexion in very young children may improve over several years. Ulnar neuropathy, believed to be the result of an ulnar shift, which narrows to the cubital tunnel, compressing the nerve against the epicondyle, has been reported in cubitus varus.[1] Other reports have noted late lateral condyle fractures,[2,3] posterolateral rotatory instability,[4] and failure of active extension.[5]

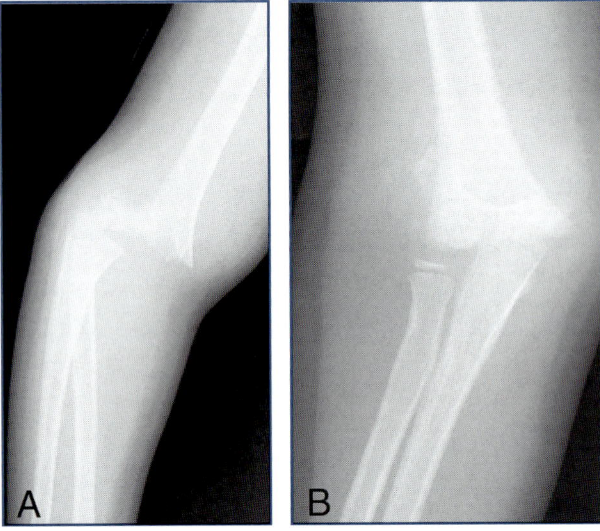

Figure 1 Example case: AP **(A)** and lateral **(B)** radiographs of a type III supracondylar humerus fracture at presentation show posteromedial displacement.

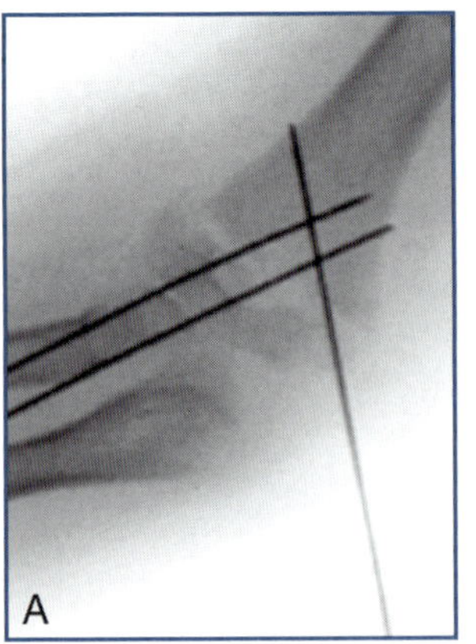

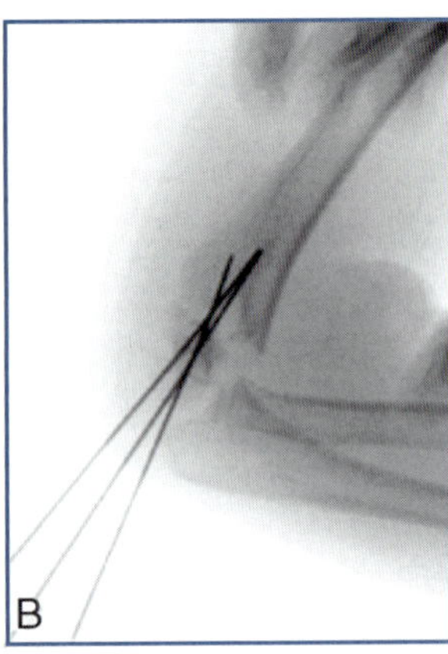

Figure 2 Example case: Intraoperative AP **(A)** and lateral **(B)** images after initial fixation. Note that the pins are small in caliber, the medial pin has no purchase on the distal fragment, and the distal fragment rotates on the pins when the surgeon attempts a lateral image. Without a good lateral image, the surgeon cannot ensure that the pins truly have purchase of both fragments.

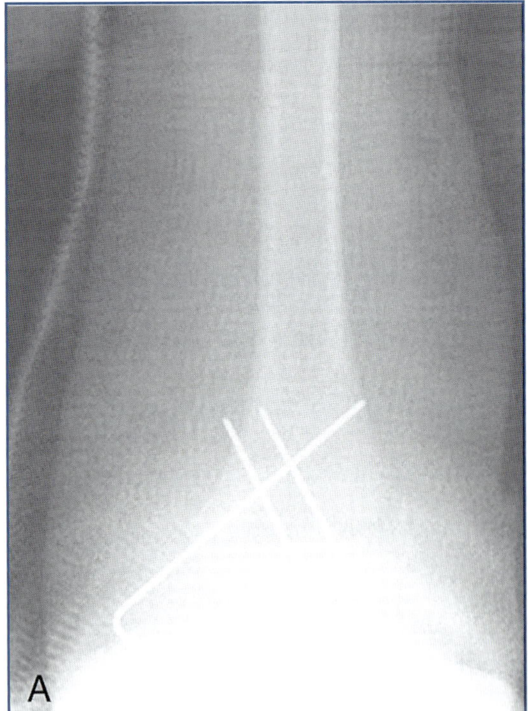

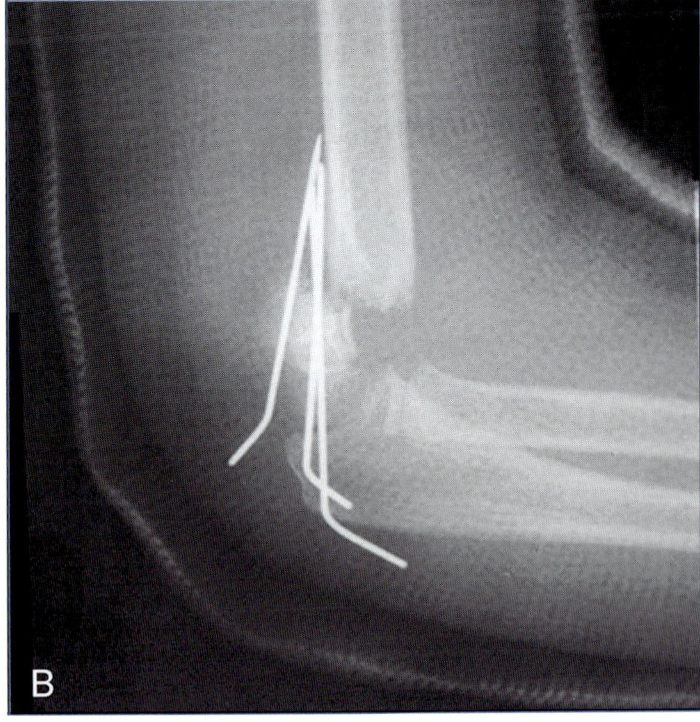

Figure 3 Example case: AP **(A)** and lateral **(B)** radiographs in the cast at 1-week follow-up demonstrate a complete loss of fixation.

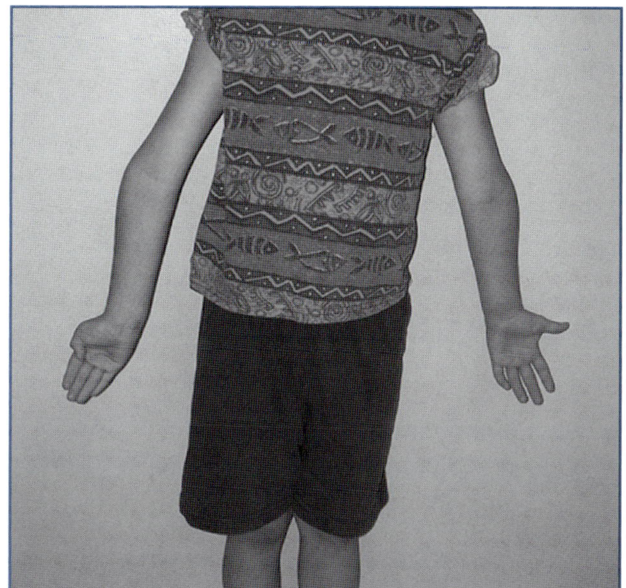

Figure 4 Example case: Cubitus varus deformity of the right arm.

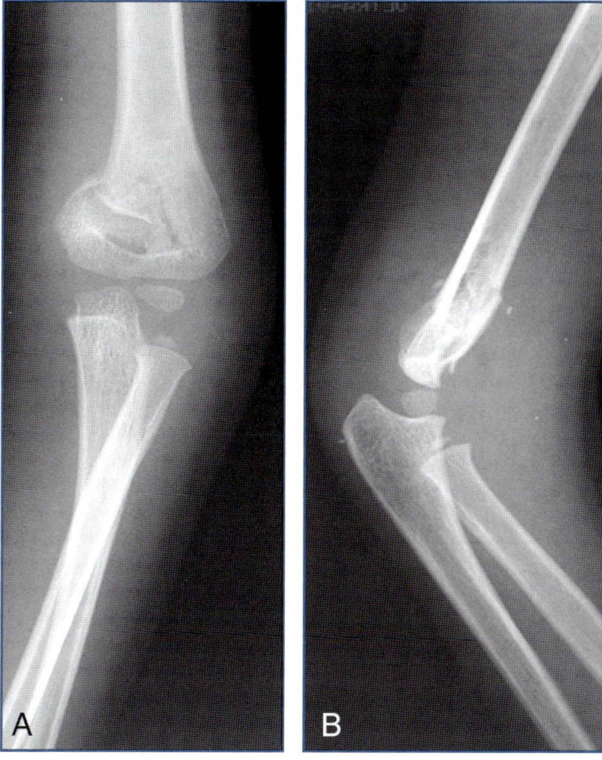

Figure 5 AP **(A)** and lateral **(B)** radiographs showing a type II supracondylar fracture of the humerus with medial impaction.

Three different clinical scenarios may lead to this problem: unrecognized varus impaction, inadequate reduction, and failure of fixation. The first scenario involves a failure to recognize a Gartland type II supracondylar humeral fracture[6] that is either unstable or has medial impaction (Figure 5). In this clinical scenario, an apparently innocuous fracture heals after 3 weeks of casting. Then, over the next several weeks, as the child regains elbow extension, it becomes apparent that the fracture has healed with varus and extension. A second scenario is failure of adequate reduction. The third scenario that leads to malunion after supracondylar humeral fracture is a loss of fixation, as illustrated in the case example.

Management of Supracondylar Humerus Fracture Malunion

The varus deformity, or varus and extension, can be corrected with an osteotomy. The goal of the osteotomy is to restore a more normal relationship between the elbow articular surface and the humeral shaft. The family should be counseled that the risks of complications with these procedures, such as loss of reduction or fixation, elbow stiffness, and neuromuscular injury, have been reported to be as high as 25%.[7] Many different techniques have been recommended, including a distal lateral closing wedge osteotomy, a three-dimensional dome osteotomy, or a medially based closing wedge osteotomy with external fixation.[8-13] The timing of the osteotomy is elective, and the osteotomy can be performed at any age.

In younger children, a relatively simple distal and laterally based closing wedge osteotomy with pin fixation and postoperative casting is recommended. In older children with more significant deformities, an osteotomy that corrects both varus and extension with more substantial fixation (screw or plates) may be warranted. In either case, preoperative template planning with true AP radiographs centered at the distal humerus is important. Longer radiographs that show most of the humerus and all of the forearm and, possibly, a comparison radiograph of the opposite elbow and arm may be helpful.

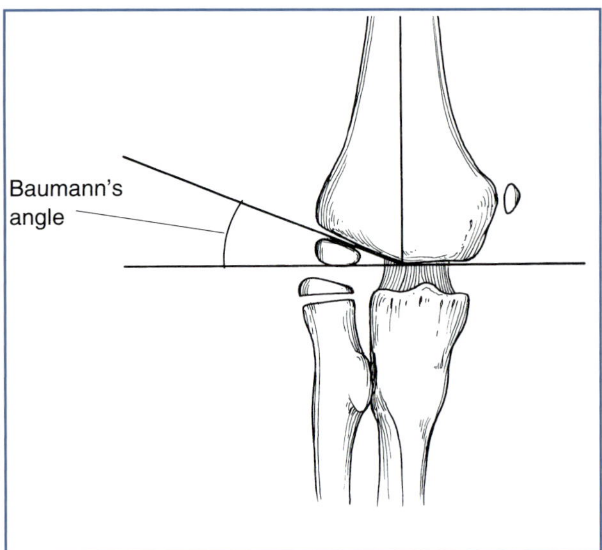

Figure 6 Baumann's angle is the angle created by the intersection of the capitellar physeal line and a line drawn along the long axis of the humerus. (Reproduced with permission from Skaggs DL: Elbow fractures in children. *J Am Acad Orthop Surg* 1997;5: 303-312.)

Preventing Supracondylar Humerus Fracture Malunion

To prevent malunion resulting from unrecognized varus impaction, it is important to obtain initial true AP and lateral radiographs. Special attention should be given to the medial column in a type II supracondylar humeral fracture, looking for impaction and displacement into varus and extension. Baumann's angle has been useful in judging the relationship of the distal fracture fragment to the humeral shaft (Figure 6). There is variability in the measurement of Baumann's angle caused by specific radiographic technique and the amount of elbow extension.[14] To ensure accuracy, the radiographs should be centered on the distal humerus. The normal Baumann's angle is 73.6° for boys and 75.6° for girls.[15] This angle can vary by several degrees from child to child, so physical examination of the carrying angle of the uninjured arm is valuable. In some patients, comparison views of the uninjured arm may be warranted. After reduction and fixation, Baumann's angle should be less than 80°. Cubitus varus has been defined as a Baumann's angle greater than 83°. It is important to understand that the full extent of the deformity will not be apparent until the child regains motion several weeks after the cast is removed.

The best way to avoid failure of adequate reduction is to ensure good operating room setup and to obtain good imaging studies. In children younger than age 3 years, the arm is short, making it difficult to position the injured distal humerus to the center of the C-arm image intensifier. For these patients, use of a radiolucent hand table is valuable. For children older than age 3 years, the collection end of the C-arm image intensifier is used as the operating table. The patient should be moved as close to the edge of the operating room table as possible, and the C-arm should be brought up tightly against the side of the table and raised to a comfortable working height for the surgeon. The monitor should be positioned against the opposite side of the table so it is within clear view. The center of the draped collection end of the C-arm image intensifier can be marked so that the elbow is brought to the center for each image, avoiding excessive images that are on the edge of the machine.

For reduction, the fracture site is first gently milked to remove interposed soft tissue. Next, gentle traction is applied to the elbow, varus and valgus malalignments are corrected, and then the elbow is placed into full flexion. To obtain a lateral image without losing reduction, the entire humerus and forearm are carefully externally rotated together in full flexion. With very unstable fractures, the C-arm itself can be rotated, rather than the arm. Generally, one or two lateral pins can be placed while obtaining the Jones image (anterior view posterior of the distal humerus in full elbow flexion). This initial fixation usually provides enough stability so that the arm can again be rotated externally to assess stability and reduction. In the rare instances in which soft tissue cannot be milked out of the fracture site to obtain a satisfactory closed reduction, open reduction is necessary.

The keys to avoiding and addressing loss of fixation include proper pinning technique, postpinning intraoperative evaluation for fracture stability, and early postoperative follow-up in very unstable fractures. Optimal pin fixation in supracondylar humeral fractures is a frequently studied and debated issue. The standard has been crossed-pin fixation, using both medial and lateral entry pins. This fixation may be best for very unstable fractures, especially if the

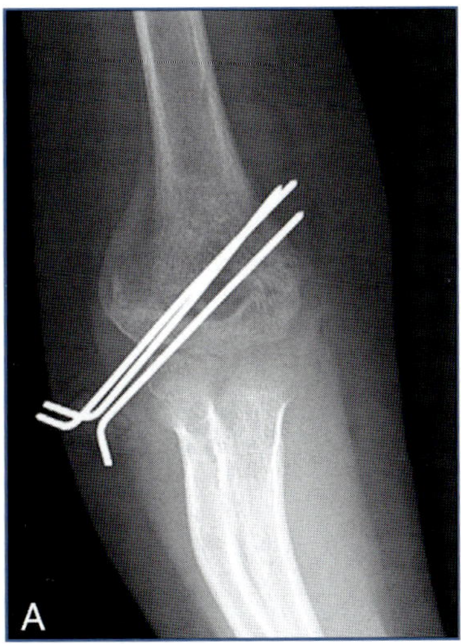

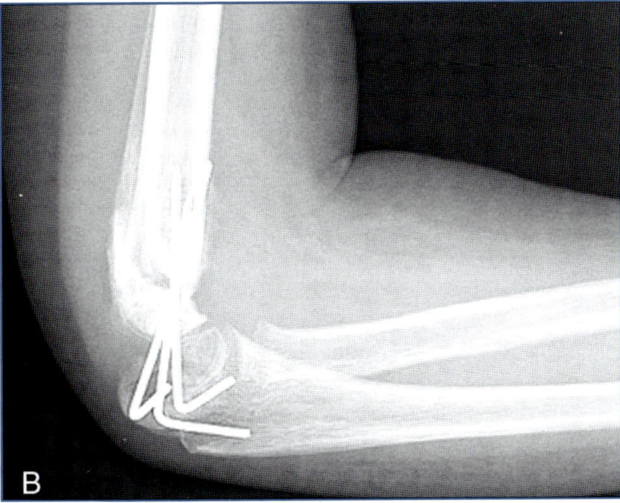

Figure 7 Example case: AP **(A)** and lateral **(B)** radiographs obtained 3 weeks after intraoperative removal of the initial pins, repeat reduction, and repinning. Note that both extension and varus were corrected, but 5 mm of lateral translation was accepted without opening the fracture. Ideally, the lateral pins should have a more divergent configuration.

fracture line on the lateral side is very low, making multiple lateral pins difficult. To avoid ulnar nerve injury or irritation with a medial pin, many proponents of this technique recommend a 5-mm incision. The surgeon spreads down to the medial epicondyle, protects the ulnar nerve posteriorly, and places the medial pin.

After reports of iatrogenic ulnar nerve injuries, there are an increasing number of proponents of lateral-entry pinning for most or all supracondylar fractures of the humerus.[16-18] The most stable lateral pin fixation involves a divergent configuration.[19] If the fracture remains unstable after two divergent lateral pins, a third lateral pin can be added. Regardless of pin technique, the surgeon should ensure that each pin has satisfactory purchase on both the distal fragment and the humeral shaft (Figure 2). Lateral entry pins should have purchase of the medial column as well. One of the most common errors is pin placement that is too anterior or posterior, missing a small distal fragment. If good intraoperative images are not obtained, inadequate fixation may be overlooked.

In loss of fixation, the distal fragment is often fixed by only one pin. The fragment then rotates on this pin; this rotation is not noted until the child returns for postoperative radiographs, and the radiology technician rotates the cast to get radiographs of the distal humerus. To ensure stability, it is valuable to gently stress the fracture site after pinning. The elbow can be taken through a gentle range of flexion, extension, and rotation. Images from the C-arm image intensifier after this stress test are compared to immediate post-pinning images to determine whether there is any change in position. If there is a change in position, then the fixation is unsatisfactory. One or more pins may need to be replaced or reoriented. Adding a third pin may solve the problem. In very unstable fractures, follow-up radiographs within the first week are valuable to ensure that reduction has not been lost.

Case Management and Outcome Summary

The patient was returned to the operating room the next day, and the fracture was evaluated with the C-arm image intensifier. There was early callus, but the extension and varus deformity could be corrected. Holding the correction, pin fixation was used. The elbow was then taken through a range of motion, and the fixation was found to be stable. The arm was placed in a cast. Pins were removed 3 weeks later (Figure 7). Follow-up radiographs at 6 months show a healed fracture in satisfactory position (Figure 8).

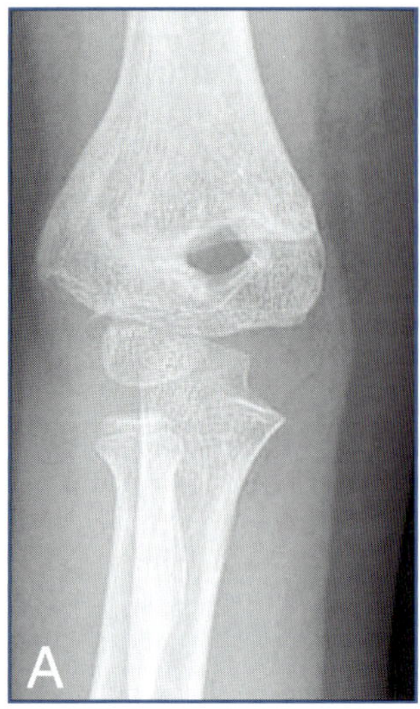

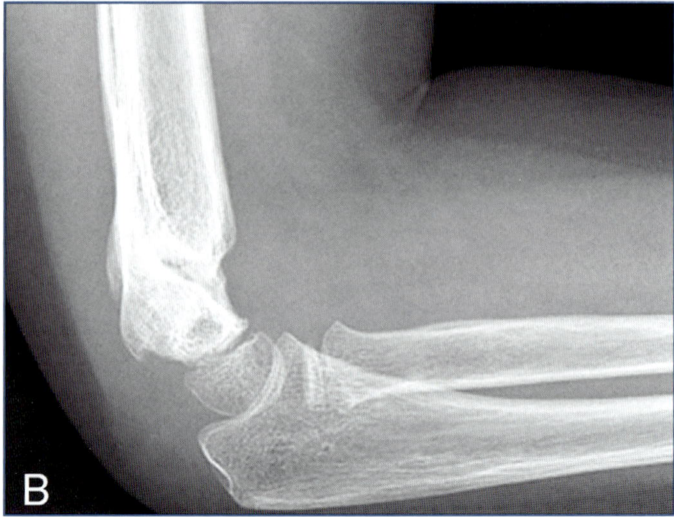

Figure 8 Example case: At 6-month follow-up, AP **(A)** and lateral **(B)** radiographs show healing in good alignment. The child had a normal range of motion, a normal carrying angle, and no other symptoms.

Strategies to Avoid Common Complications

In the case presented here, the fracture was rotationally unstable, and initial fixation was unsatisfactory. The inadequacy of this fixation was not recognized in the operating room. Fortunately, the loss of the fixation was recognized at a follow-up within the first week. Revision pinning led to a good result.

A clinically important malunion after supracondylar humeral fracture, which is both cosmetically unacceptable and functionally disabling, is uncommon in the current era of high-quality imaging and a technique of closed reduction and percutaneous pinning. This complication can occur from misjudgment of the fracture, inadequate reduction, or inadequate pin fixation.

References

1. Abe M, Ishizu T, Shirai H, et al: Tardy ulnar nerve palsy caused by cubitus varus deformity. *J Hand Surg [Am]* 1995;20:5-9.
2. Davids JR, Maguire MF, Mubarak SJ, et al: Lateral condylar fracture of the humerus following posttraumatic cubitus varus. *J Pediatr Orthop* 1994;14:466-470.
3. Takahara M, Sasaki I, Kimura T, et al: Second fracture of the distal humerus after varus malunion of a supracondylar fracture in children. *J Bone Joint Surg Br* 1998;80:791-797.
4. O'Driscoll SW, Spinner RJ, McKee MD, et al: Tardy posterolateral rotatory instability of the elbow due to cubitus varus. *J Bone Joint Surg Am* 2001;83:1358-1369.
5. Smith IJ, Williams CP: Failure of active extension after traumatic cubitus varus: A case report. *J Bone Joint Surg Br* 2002;84:1180-1182.
6. Gartland JJ: Management of supracondylar fractures of the humerus in children. *Surg Gynecol Obstet* 1959;109:145-154.
7. Beaty JH, Kasser JR: Supracondylar fractures of the distal humerus, in Rockwood CA, Wilkins KE (eds): *Fractures in Children*, ed 5. Philadelphia, PA, Lippincott-Williams & Wilkins, 2001, pp 577-624.
8. Bellemore M, Barret I, Middleton RW, et al: Supracondylar osteotomy of the humerus for correction of cubitus varus. *J Bone Joint Surg Br* 1984;66:566-572.
9. Gaddy BC, Manske PR, Pruitt DL, et al: Distal humeral osteotomy for correction of posttraumatic cubitus varus. *J Pediatr Orthop* 1994;14:214-219.
10. Graham B, Tresdwell SJ, Beauchamp RD, et al: Supracondylar osteotomy of the humerus for correction of cubitus varus. *J Pediatr Orthop* 1990;10:228-231.

11. LaBelle H, Bunnell WP, Duhaime M, et al: Cubitus varus deformity following supracondylar fractures of the humerus in children. *J Pediatr Orthop* 1982;2:539-546.
12. Sweeney JG: Osteotomy of the humerus for malunion of supracondylar fractures. *J Bone Joint Surg Br* 1975;57:117.
13. Voss FR, Kasser JR, Trepman E, et al: Uniplanar supracondylar humeral osteotomy with preset Kirschner wires for posttraumatic cubitus varus. *J Pediatr Orthop* 1994;14: 471-478.
14. Skaggs DL: Elbow fractures in children: Diagnosis and management. *J Am Acad Orthop Surg* 1997;5: 303-312.
15. Keenan WN, Clegg J: Variation of Baumann's angle with age, sex, and side: Implications for its use in radiological monitoring of supracondylar fracture of the humerus in children. *J Pediatr Orthop* 1996;16: 97-98.
16. Gordon JE, Patton CM, Luhmann SJ, et al: Fracture instability after pinning of displaced supracondylar distal humerus fractures in children. *J Pediatr Orthop* 2001;21:313-318.
17. Skaggs DL, Hale JM, Bassett J, et al: Operative treatment of supracondylar fractures of the humerus in children: The consequences of pin placement. *J Bone Joint Surg Am* 2001;83:735-740.
18. Skaggs DL, Cluck MW, Mostofi A, Flynn JM, Kay RM: Lateral-entry pin fixation in the management of supracondylar fractures in children. *J Bone Joint Surg Am* 2004;86: 702-707.
19. Lee SS, Mahar AT, Miesen D, et al: Displaced pediatric supracondylar humerus fractures: Biomechanical analysis of percutaneous pinning techniques. *J Pediatr Orthop* 2002; 22:440-443.

Chapter 8

Supracondylar Humerus Fracture With Neurovascular Compromise

John M. Flynn, MD

Case Presentation

History

A 5-year-old boy was brought in after a fall from a height onto an outstretched hand. A thorough assessment revealed that his injuries were confined to the left upper extremity. He had a very swollen left elbow with an obvious deformity, but the skin was intact. Function of his ulnar and radial nerves was normal, but his anterior interosseous nerve was injured. He could not actively flex his index finger or thumb distal interphalangeal (DIP) joint. With the arm in extension, the hand was satisfactorily perfused, but a radial pulse could not be palpated.

Initial images showed a severely displaced type III supracondylar fracture of the humerus with posterolateral displacement (Figure 1). Because of his neurovascular compromise, the patient was brought urgently to the operating room.

After the patient was anesthetized in the operating room, his left elbow was brought over the C-arm image intensifier. The anterior muscle mass of the upper arm was gently manipulated in an effort to milk the entrapped soft tissues out of the fracture site. The deformity at the elbow improved, and the skin tenting resolved. With the elbow extended, the valgus malalignment was corrected, and the standard reduction maneuver was performed, flexing the elbow with manipulative pressure on the distal fragment.

Current Problem and Treatment

The surgeon immediately recognized that anatomic reduction could not be obtained. This was particularly evident on the lateral view. Findings suggested that interposed tissue within the fracture site precluded reduction. With each attempt to flex the elbow, the patient's distal forearm and hand became pale, raising concern that the interposed tissue included the brachial artery. Based on these observations, a decision was made to perform an open reduction before fixation.

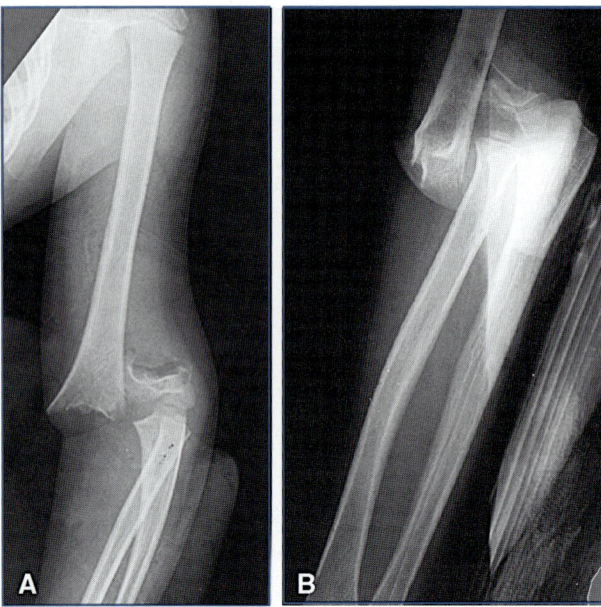

Figure 1 Example case: AP **(A)** and lateral **(B)** radiographs show a type III supracondylar fracture of the humerus with posterolateral displacement.

Discussion

Recognizing the Problem and Situations at High Risk

Neurovascular compromise occurs with alarming frequency in association with severely displaced pediatric elbow fractures.[1-3] It is estimated that 10% to 20% of type III supracondylar humerus fractures have an absent pulse.[4] The injury to the brachial artery is at the fracture site, making angiography and other methods to locate the source of the problem unnecessary in the initial evaluation. Because the pediatric elbow has substantial collateral circulation, the absence of a palpable pulse is less important than the integrity of the distal perfusion.

Neurologic injuries also occur with some frequency after supracondylar humerus fractures. The incidence of nerve injury ranges from 10% to 49% in different series.[5,6] The anterior interosseous nerve, which appears to be injured most commonly,[5,6] can be tested by asking the child to flex the thumb and index finger DIP joint. With posterolateral fracture displacement, the neurovascular bundle is stretched over the metaphysis of the distal humerus, making median nerve or anterior interosseous nerve injury most likely. In posteromedial fracture displacement, the radial nerve is stretched over the lateral distal humeral metaphysis. Ulnar nerve injury is most common in flexion-type supracondylar humerus fractures. In posteromedial fracture displacement (about 75% of cases), the radial nerve is at risk; in posterolateral fractures, the brachial artery and median nerve are at risk.

Management of Supracondylar Humerus Fractures

Children with severely displaced supracondylar humerus fractures and vascular compromise typically present with one of two different scenarios: (1) the hand is perfused but the radial pulse is absent, or (2) the hand is white and not perfused (rare). Thus, neurologic function, distal pulses, and perfusion should be evaluated immediately on presentation (Figure 2).

A gentle partial reduction of the fracture under conscious sedation in the emergency department is reasonable if the skin is threatened and immediate surgery is not possible. This initial, gentle maneuver may take some of the tension off the stretched neurovascular structures. The fracture is then splinted in 30° of extension, and plans should be made for immediate surgery.

In the operating room, the child is anesthetized, and if an anatomic reduction can be obtained, the fracture is stabilized with percutaneous pins (usually two or three lateral entry pins or crossed medial and lateral entry pins if necessary), and distal perfusion is reassessed. Inability to obtain anatomic reduction may indicate that the brachial artery is entrapped (as in this case). The fracture should be opened when soft tissues cannot be removed from the fracture site with gentle milking maneuvers.[7]

When closed reduction and percutaneous pinning are performed, the vascular status of the hand should be monitored carefully. If the pulse is palpable and the hand well perfused, the arm should be splinted in 30° of extension, and the child should be observed as an inpatient for at least 24 hours. If the pulse is not palpable but can be detected by Doppler evaluation, the child's arm should be splinted in about 30° of flexion and observed closely in the early postoperative period, with a plan to return to the operating room immedi-

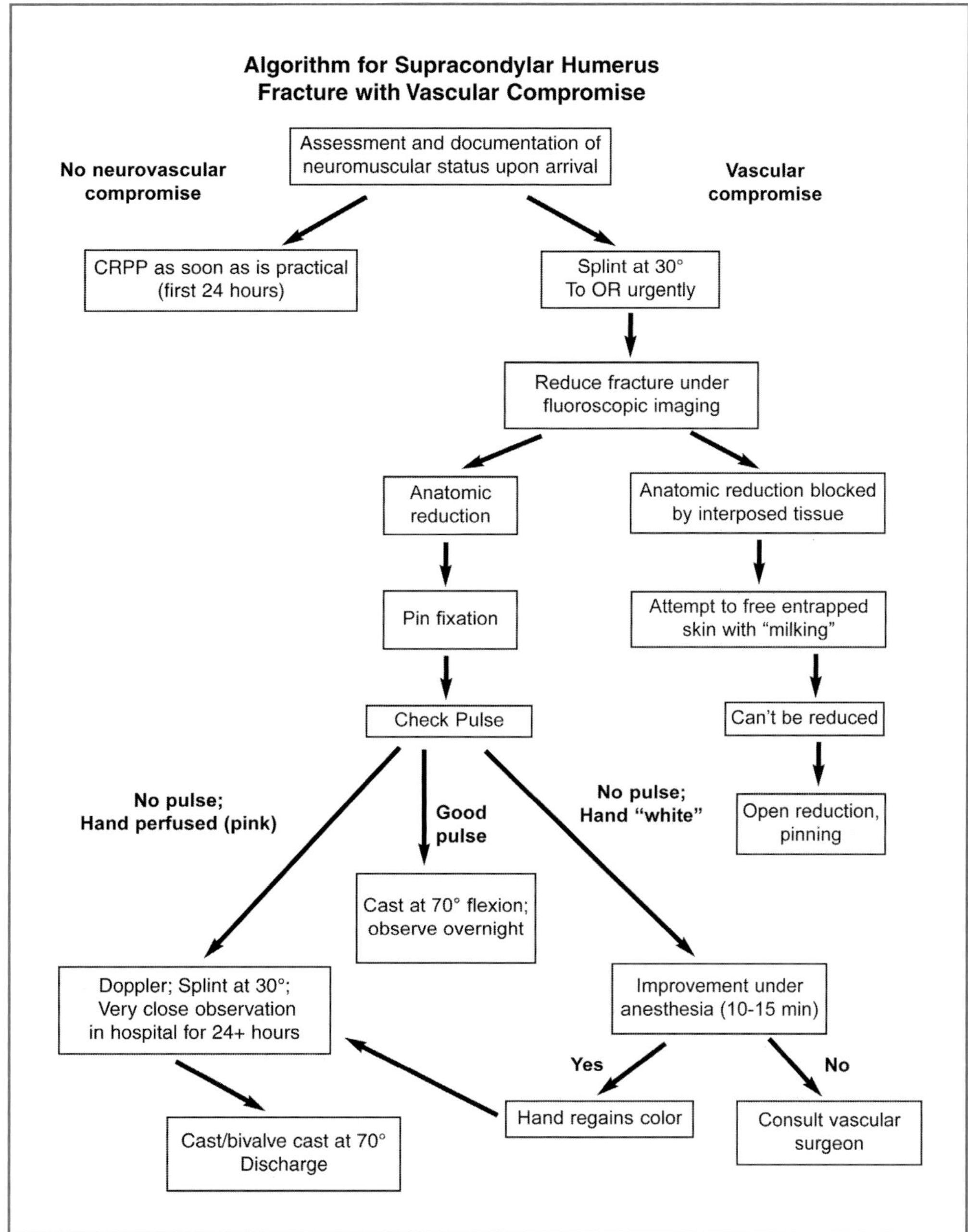

Figure 2 Algorithm for supracondylar humeral fracture with vascular compromise.

ately if there is severe pain, paresthesias, or any sign of vascular compromise or compartment syndrome.

When the pulse is not palpable and not detectable by Doppler evaluation, the child should be observed while under anesthesia for 10 to 15 minutes because a detectable pulse returns in many instances. If there is no improvement in 10 to 15 minutes, the vascular team should be consulted because exploration and vascular repair may be warranted. This scenario is quite unusual.

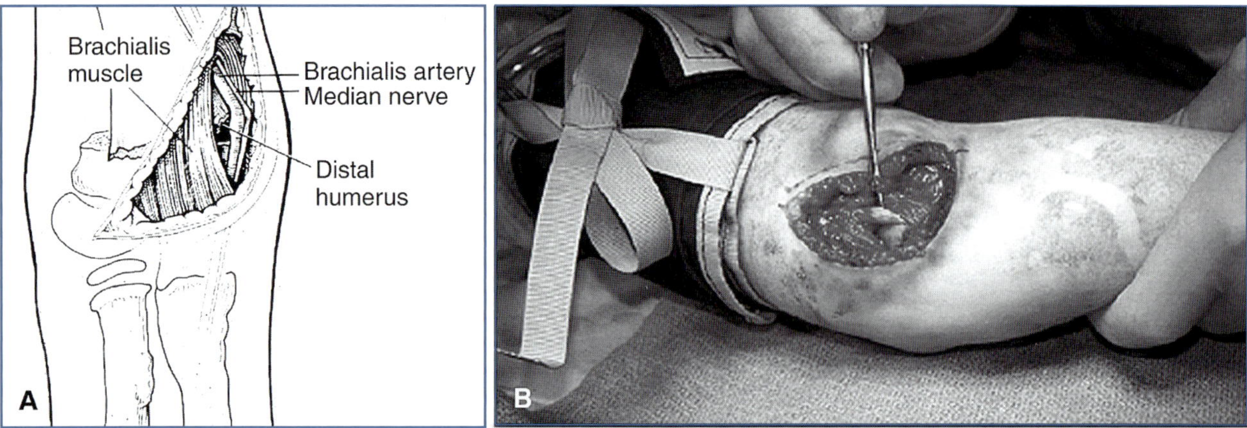

Figure 3 A, Proper location for incision to open a supracondylar fracture of the humerus. In most cases, the surgeon will find a large tear in the brachialis muscle, and the brachial artery and median nerve are just below the skin, draped over the displaced humeral metaphysis. (Reproduced with permission from Kasser JR, Beaty JH: Supracondylar fractures of the distal humerus, in Beaty JH, Kasser JR (eds) *Rockwood and Wilkins' Fractures in Children,* ed 5. Philadelphia, PA, Lippincott-Williams & Wilkins, 2001, pp 577-624.) **B,** Example case: In this intraoperative photograph, the surgeon has exposed the fracture site and has located the neurovascular bundle, which was trapped in the fracture.

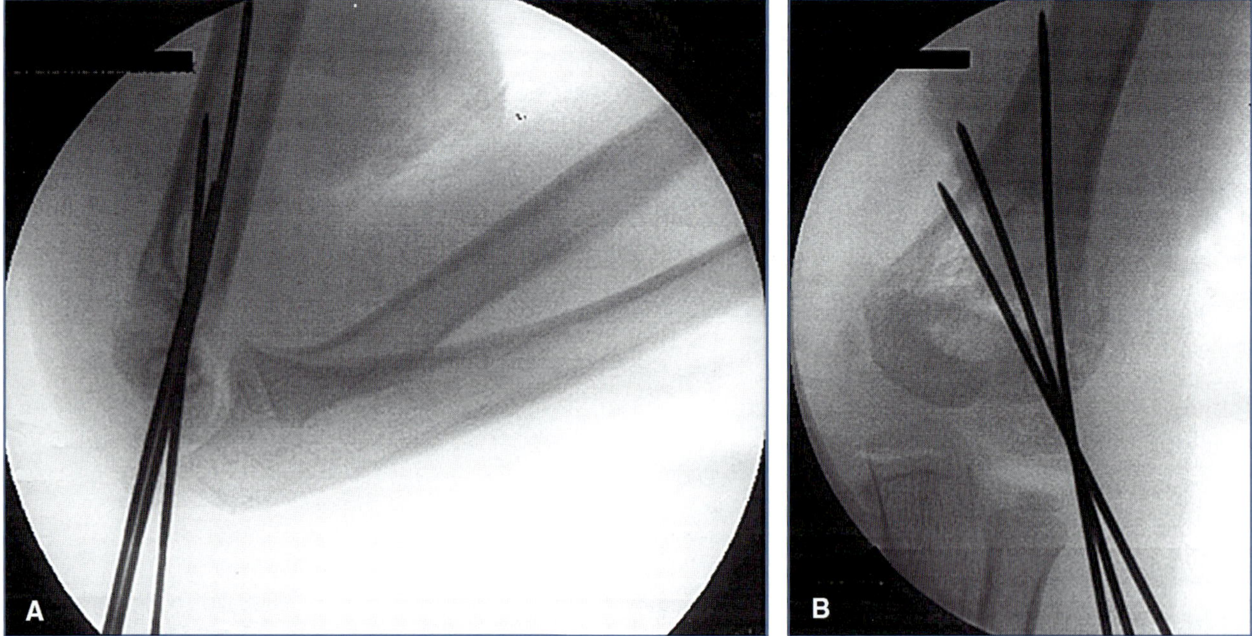

Figure 4 Example case: Intraoperative AP **(A)** and lateral **(B)** images after pinning and range of motion. Alignment is satisfactory, although the distal fragment was fixed in slight valgus and extension. Fixation was stable.

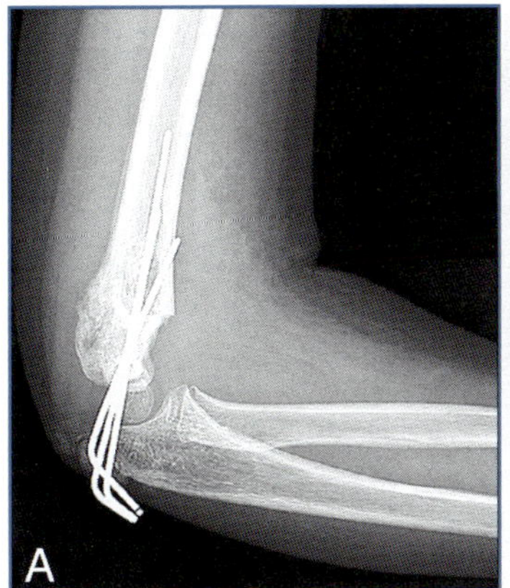

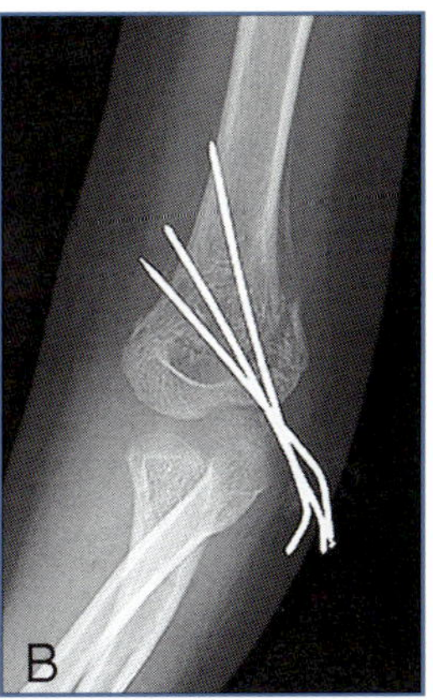

Figure 5 Example case: AP **(A)** and lateral **(B)** radiographs of the distal humerus obtained 3 weeks after pinning show that fixation was maintained and that there is enough healing to allow pin removal.

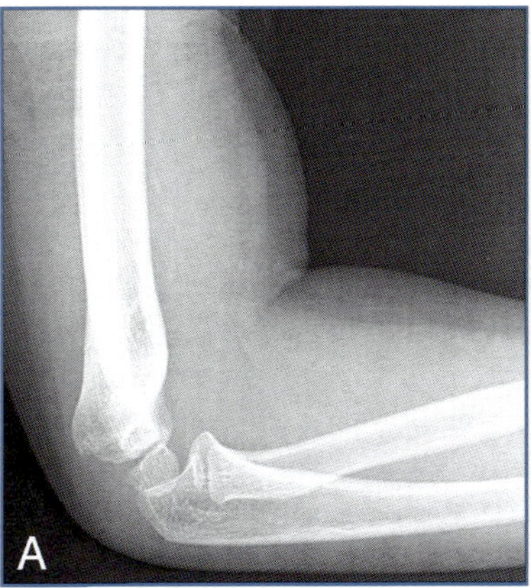

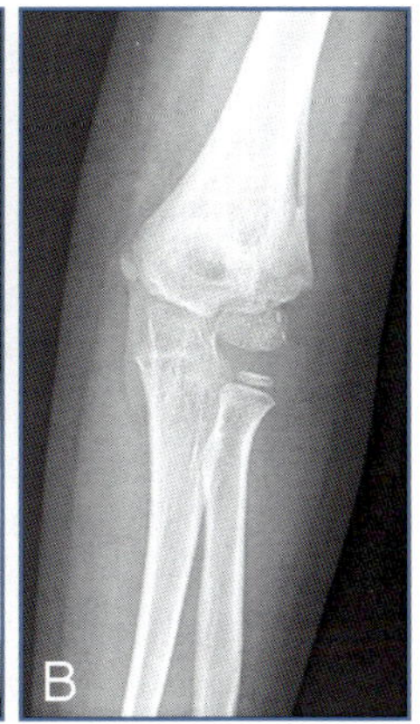

Figure 6 Example case: AP **(A)** and lateral **(B)** radiographs 5 months after injury. Range of motion has returned to normal; remodeling at the fracture site continues.

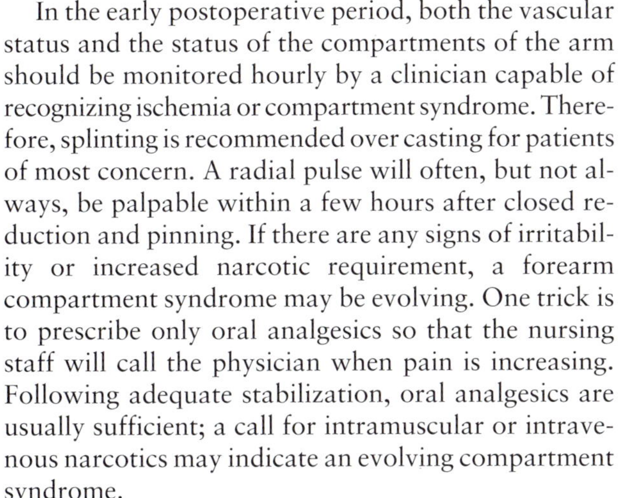

In the early postoperative period, both the vascular status and the status of the compartments of the arm should be monitored hourly by a clinician capable of recognizing ischemia or compartment syndrome. Therefore, splinting is recommended over casting for patients of most concern. A radial pulse will often, but not always, be palpable within a few hours after closed reduction and pinning. If there are any signs of irritability or increased narcotic requirement, a forearm compartment syndrome may be evolving. One trick is to prescribe only oral analgesics so that the nursing staff will call the physician when pain is increasing. Following adequate stabilization, oral analgesics are usually sufficient; a call for intramuscular or intravenous narcotics may indicate an evolving compartment syndrome.

One pitfall is the child with a median nerve injury at the time of fracture. These patients have reduced sensation in the forearm, and a compartment syndrome can develop with very little pain. If the forearm feels tense, compartment pressures should be measured. Prior to discharge from the hospital, most surgeons place the arm in a cast or a bivalve cast. Pins are typically removed at 3 weeks. Families should be advised that it may take up to 6 months for motion to be fully restored. Complete return of motion is likely if the reduction is satisfactory.

Neurologic injuries, such as the anterior interosseous nerve injury demonstrated here, should be documented and observed. Most of these injuries resolve within 4 months. If significant motor deficit exists after 4 months, electromyography and nerve conduction velocity studies may be appropriate.

Preventing Neurovascular Compromise in Supracondylar Humerus Fractures

Preventing neurovascular problems after supracondylar humerus fractures requires a high index of suspicion, especially in type III fractures. It is important to understand that neurovascular injuries are quite common in the most displaced fractures. Therefore, preoperative neurovascular status should be carefully documented. If the hand is not well perfused and/or the pulse is not detectable on Doppler evaluation, and the fracture has been adequately reduced and fixed, a vascular specialist should be consulted. If the hand is well perfused but a radial pulse cannot be palpated, the arm should be splinted in about 30° of elbow flexion and no tight circular bandages used. Intravenous narcotics should be avoided until the patient is awake and can be evaluated by an experienced surgeon. This evaluation should be followed with repeat evaluation by a reliable observer, with special attention to the possibility of evolving compartment syndrome.

Case Management and Outcome Summary

A sterile tourniquet was placed high on the patient's left arm after the arm was prepped and draped. After the tourniquet was inflated, a gently curved incision was made on the anterior medial aspect of the distal arm, centered on the area of skin that had been tented (Figure 3). There was a large tear in the brachialis muscle. The median nerve was identified and protected. The fracture site was exposed through the brachialis tear. The brachial artery was folded into the fracture site but not disrupted. The artery was then freed, along with some periosteum and brachialis muscle. The fracture was then easily reducible. After placement of three divergent lateral pins, the elbow was taken through a range of motion with fluoroscopic imaging and found to be completely stable (Figure 4). After fixation, perfusion in the hand was reassessed. The hand was now pink, and although the radial pulse could not be palpated, a pulse could be detected by Doppler evaluation.

The wound was closed in layers with bioabsorbable sutures, the pins were cut and bent, and Xeroform (Tyco Healthcare Group, Mansfield, MA) was wrapped around the base to prevent the pins from migrating under the skin. By the time the closure was complete, a faintly palpable radial pulse could be felt.

The patient's elbow and forearm were splinted in about 30° of flexion, with a window to visualize the hand and palpate the radial pulse. He was observed as an inpatient for 36 hours; then his elbow and forearm were placed in a long arm cast with 70° of elbow flexion, and he was discharged. The pins were removed at 3 weeks (Figure 5). Although full extension and full elbow flexion were restored, the pace of the patient's improvement was much slower than is typical for fractures treated with closed management.

At 5-month follow-up, the fracture was healed in a satisfactory position (Figure 6). He had no pain, his range of motion was 0° to 140°, and he had a normal carrying angle. He did have some widening of his scar medially but had no complaints. The outcome was good.

Strategies to Avoid Common Complications

In this case, recognizing an inadequate reduction in the face of vascular compromise led to open reduction, release of an entrapped brachial artery, and stable pinning (Figure 2).

References

1. Copley LA, Dormans JP, Davidson RS: Vascular injuries and their sequelae in pediatric supracondylar humeral fractures: Toward a goal of prevention. *J Pediatr Orthop* 1996; 16:99-103.
2. Shaw BA, Kasser JR, Emans JB, et al: Management of vascular injuries in displaced supracondylar humerus fractures without arteriography. *J Orthop Trauma* 1990;4:25-29.
3. Flynn JM, Sarwark JF, Waters PM, et al: The operative management of pediatric fractures of the upper extremity. *J Bone Joint Surg Am* 2002;84:2078-2089.
4. Kasser JR, Beaty JH: Supracondylar fractures of the distal humerus, in Beaty JH, Kasser JR (eds): *Rockwood and Wilkins' Fractures in Children*, ed 5. Philadelphia, PA, Lippincott-Williams & Wilkins, 2001, pp 577-624.
5. Mehlman CT, Crawford AH, McMillion TL, et al: Operative treatment of supracondylar fractures of the humerus in children: The Cincinnati experience. *Acta Orthop Belg* 1996;62(suppl 1):41-50.
6. Campbell CC, Waters PM, Emans JB, et al: Neurovascular injury and displacement in type III supracondylar humerus fractures. *J Pediatr Orthop* 1995;15:47-52.
7. Archibeck MJ, Scott SM, Peters CL: Brachialis muscle entrapment in displaced supracondylar humerus fractures: A technique of closed reduction and report of initial results. *J Pediatr Orthop* 1997;17: 298-302.

Chapter 9

Irreducible Fracture of the Proximal Humerus

John M. Flynn, MD

Case Presentation

History

A right-handed 15-year-old high school quarterback who fell directly onto his shoulder when he was tackled during a game reported hearing a "snap," followed by immediate shoulder pain. He was taken to an emergency department where radiographs showed a displaced Salter-Harris type II proximal humerus fracture. His neurovascular examination was normal, and no other injuries were noted.

Initial management consisted of closed reduction under conscious sedation. The initial treating orthopaedist reported that the reduction was difficult, but that satisfactory alignment was obtained. The patient's arm was placed in a coaptation splint with a sling and swathe.

Current Problem and Treatment

The patient's family sought a second opinion 2 days after the injury because they were concerned about the appearance of the postreduction radiographs. Repeat radiographs of the arm in the coaptation splint were obtained, showing significant angulation and displacement. The family was counseled extensively on the excellent remodeling potential of the proximal humerus. In an attempt to improve the shortening, the coaptation splint was exchanged for a hanging arm cast, and the family was asked to return at 1 week after injury. Radiographs obtained 1 week after the injury showed little improvement (Figure 1), specifically there was shortening, 100% translation, and 70° of angulation.

Discussion

Recognizing the Problem and Situations at High Risk

Proximal humeral fractures are relatively rare injuries in children, comprising about 5% of pediatric fractures. Proximal humeral physeal injuries, as in this case, are even more unusual, comprising less than 1% of pediatric fractures. Because of the range of motion of the proximal humerus and the rapid growth present at the proximal humeral physis, these injuries have a reputation for

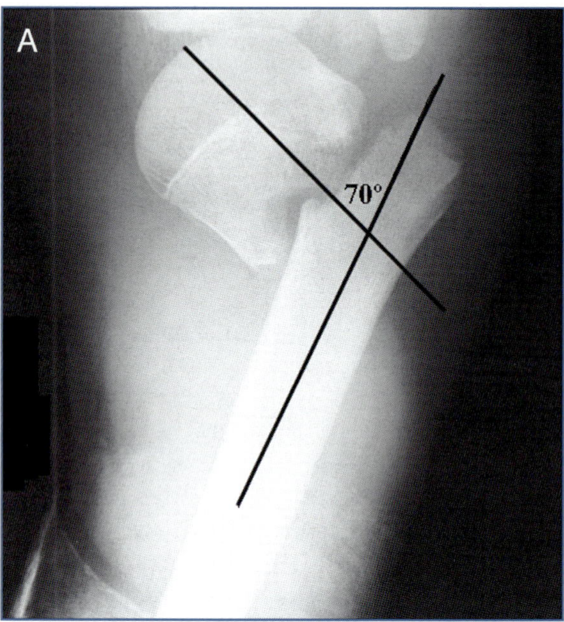

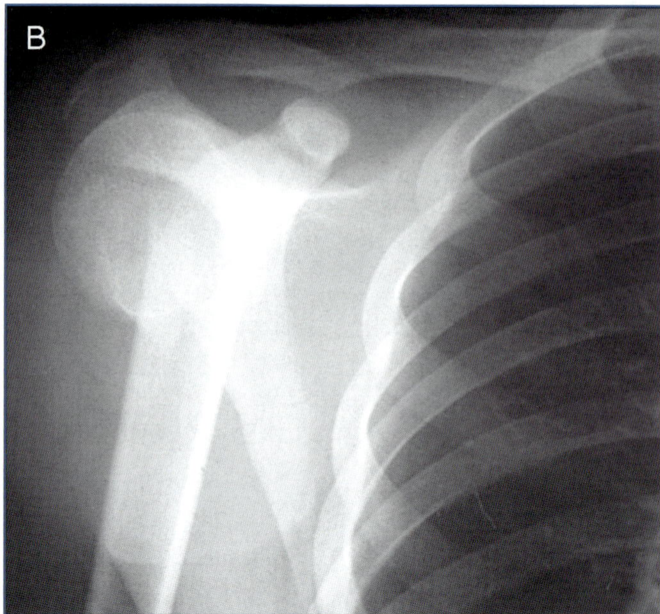

Figure 1 Example case: AP **(A)** and lateral **(B)** radiographs of the proximal humerus obtained 1 week after injury while the patient was being treated with a hanging cast. Note the shortening, 100% translation, and 70° of angulation at the fracture site.

extraordinary remodeling potential. Therefore, the vast majority of displaced proximal humeral fractures should be treated with immobilization.

Blount[1] said, "The greatest fallacy is to think that accurate reduction of an epiphyseal fracture at the proximal end of the humerus is important enough to require open reduction." Discussion of a proximal humeral fracture belongs in this text because there are some specific indications for reduction (with or without fixation). A dogmatic approach that supports accepting any amount of deformity will lead to some unsatisfactory functional results. Reduction is advised in three specific scenarios: (1) severe deformity with tented skin or an open fracture, or neurovascular compromise; (2) a completely displaced Salter-Harris type I fracture in an infant; and (3) unacceptable alignment in an adolescent. This final indication, illustrated in the case presentation, is the most controversial.

Management of Proximal Humerus Fractures

The controversy regarding the need for reduction is illustrated by findings reported in two recent clinical series. Beringer and associates[2] evaluated 21 patients (mean age, 14.1 years) who sustained a proximal humerus fracture at least 4 years prior to the study. Of these 21 patients, 12 had mild pain, weakness, or motion loss. Several had humeral shortening or imperfect radiographic remodeling, but these findings did not seem to correlate with clinical outcome. Most fractures were managed by closed means and had no complications. Nine patients had some form of surgical intervention, and three of these nine had a complication. The authors concluded that their study supported previous recommendations to avoid surgical intervention. Dobbs and associates[3] reported on 28 patients, 19 of whom were age 15 years or older. Of these 28 patients, 25 had reduction and fixation; in five patients, the reduction was blocked by periosteum or the biceps tendon. At 4-year follow-up, the patients had normal motion and no complications. These investigators emphasized that most series include only a small number of patients older than age 15 years. They concluded that it was "inappropriate to assume older adolescents with this injury will do uniformly well with nonoperative treatment."[3]

Acceptable displacement of a proximal humerus fracture is somewhat controversial. One often quoted source recommends 70° of angulation and 100% displacement in children younger than age 5 years, 40° to 70° of angulation in children ages 5 to 12 years, and up to 40° of angulation and 50% displacement in children older than age 12 years.[4]

Cases such as the one illustrated in this chapter present specific challenges. Significantly displaced fractures in teenagers, particularly those in the dominant arm of an overhead or throwing athlete, may in some cases result in loss of shoulder motion and function if allowed to heal with significant displacement. In this case, an initial closed reduction was attempted, and the arm was immobilized. Follow-up radiographs showed persistent unacceptable angulation and displacement.

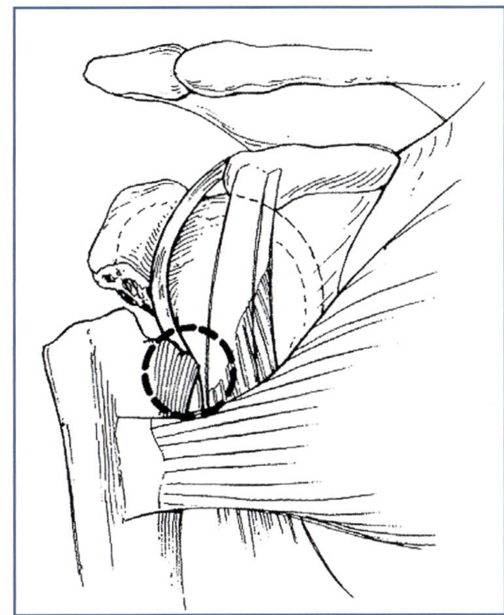

Figure 2 This diagram shows interposition of the biceps tendon between the shaft and proximal fragment of a similar fracture. (Reproduced with permission from Dobbs MB: Severely displaced proximal humeral epiphyseal fractures. *J Pediatr Orthop* 2003;23:208-215.)

Preventing Unsatisfactory Reduction in Proximal Humerus Fractures

When proposing closed reduction under anesthesia of this fracture in an adolescent, the patient and parents should be advised that open reduction may be necessary for adequate alignment, and fixation may be necessary for stabilization. In the case discussed here, interposed tissue, including the biceps tendon, blocked satisfactory reduction. These issues have been described in several studies.[3,5]

Once a satisfactory reduction is obtained, either open or closed, there are a variety of choices for internal fixation. Perhaps the most popular technique, and the one that I have used, involves inserting threaded pins through the lateral cortex of the humerus engaging the humeral head fragment. Pins can be left exposed or buried beneath the skin. Pin migration in this area is a well-reported complication. Although the risk is lower in the strong bone of an adolescent humerus compared to the osteopenic bone of an elderly adult, great care should be taken to ensure that each pin has excellent purchase in bone. I strongly recommend close follow-up with radiographs after pinning. Any pins that appear to change position should be removed immediately.

An alternative to pin fixation is elastic stable intramedullary nailing (ESIN). The French proponents of this technique have used retrograde titanium elastic nails to reduce and maintain reduction in these fractures. ESIN has several advantages, although it is technically challenging and requires incisions around the elbow as well as a possible open reduction at the shoulder. Retrograde nailing eliminates the risk of pin migration, as well as the risk of damage to the biceps tendon and neurovascular structures by misplaced threaded proximal humerus pins.

Case Management and Outcome Summary

The patient's fracture had displaced beyond accepted standards for his age group, and his family was concerned about the loss of motion from malunion. Thus, a decision was made to proceed with repeat closed reduction and possible open reduction with fixation.

The patient was taken to the operating room, where he was positioned supine with his shoulder over a radiolucent table extension. The C-arm image intensifier was brought into position, and a closed reduction was attempted. The first maneuver, shoulder abduction in flexion, did not result in a satisfactory

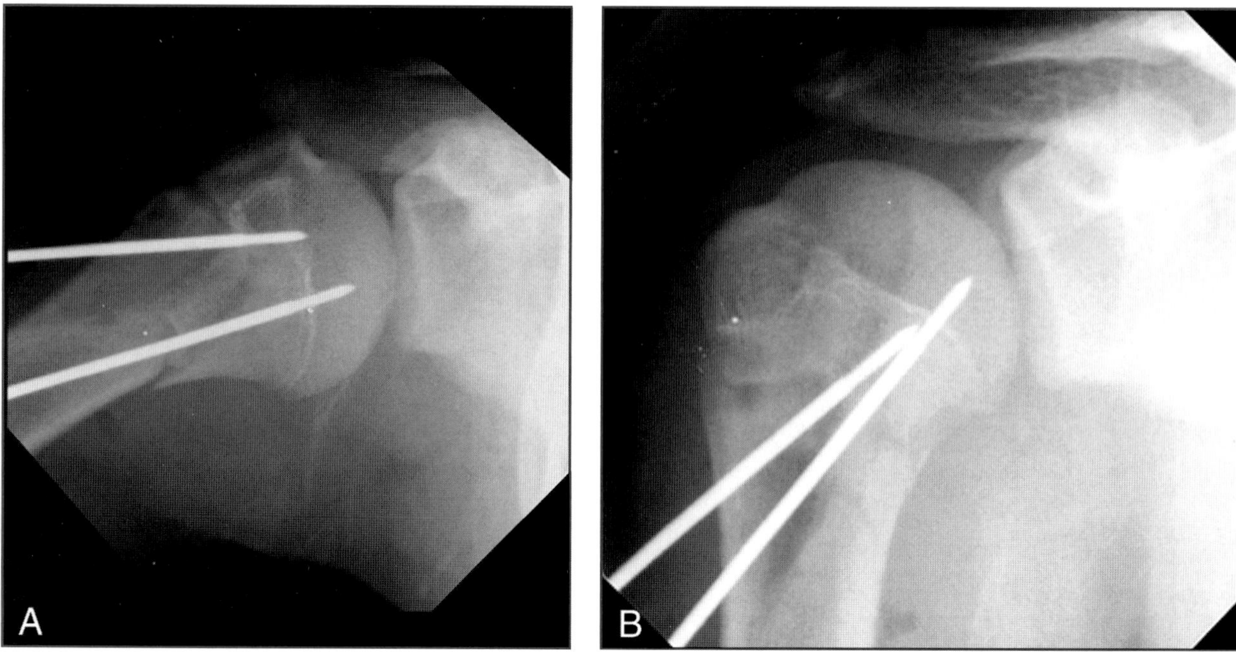

Figure 3 Example case: AP **(A)** and lateral **(B)** radiographs taken intraoperatively after open reduction and fixation of the fracture. Two partially threaded pins are holding the reduction.

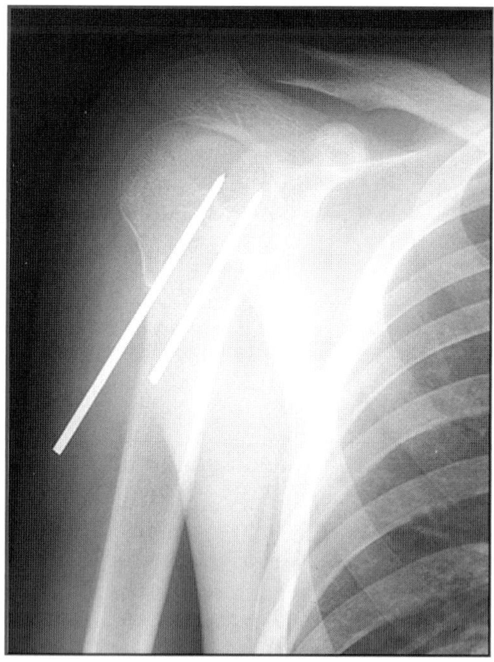

Figure 4 Example case: AP radiograph of the right humerus taken 5 weeks after surgery and just before pin removal shows healing in good position with no displacement since surgical fixation.

reduction. A second attempt, using direct manipulation in full abduction, also failed to achieve satisfactory alignment. It became obvious that interposed tissue was blocking reduction and that an open reduction was needed to achieve satisfactory alignment for pinning.

The shoulder was prepped and draped. The deltopectoral interval was used to approach the proximal humerus. The shaft fragment was found to be buttonholed partially through the deltoid muscle, and the biceps tendon was interposed between the proximal humeral fragment and the humeral shaft (Figure 2). The interposed tissue was freed, and the shaft was extricated from the deltoid. With the fragments held reduced, two pins with threaded tips were driven distal to proximal across the fracture and into the humeral epiphysis (Figure 3). Fixation was satisfactory, and stability was confirmed with a gentle range of motion of the shoulder under fluoroscopic imaging. The pins were cut short, and the skin was closed over them. The arm was placed in a swing and swath, and the fracture healed without further displacement (Figure 4). The pins were removed 6 weeks later. The

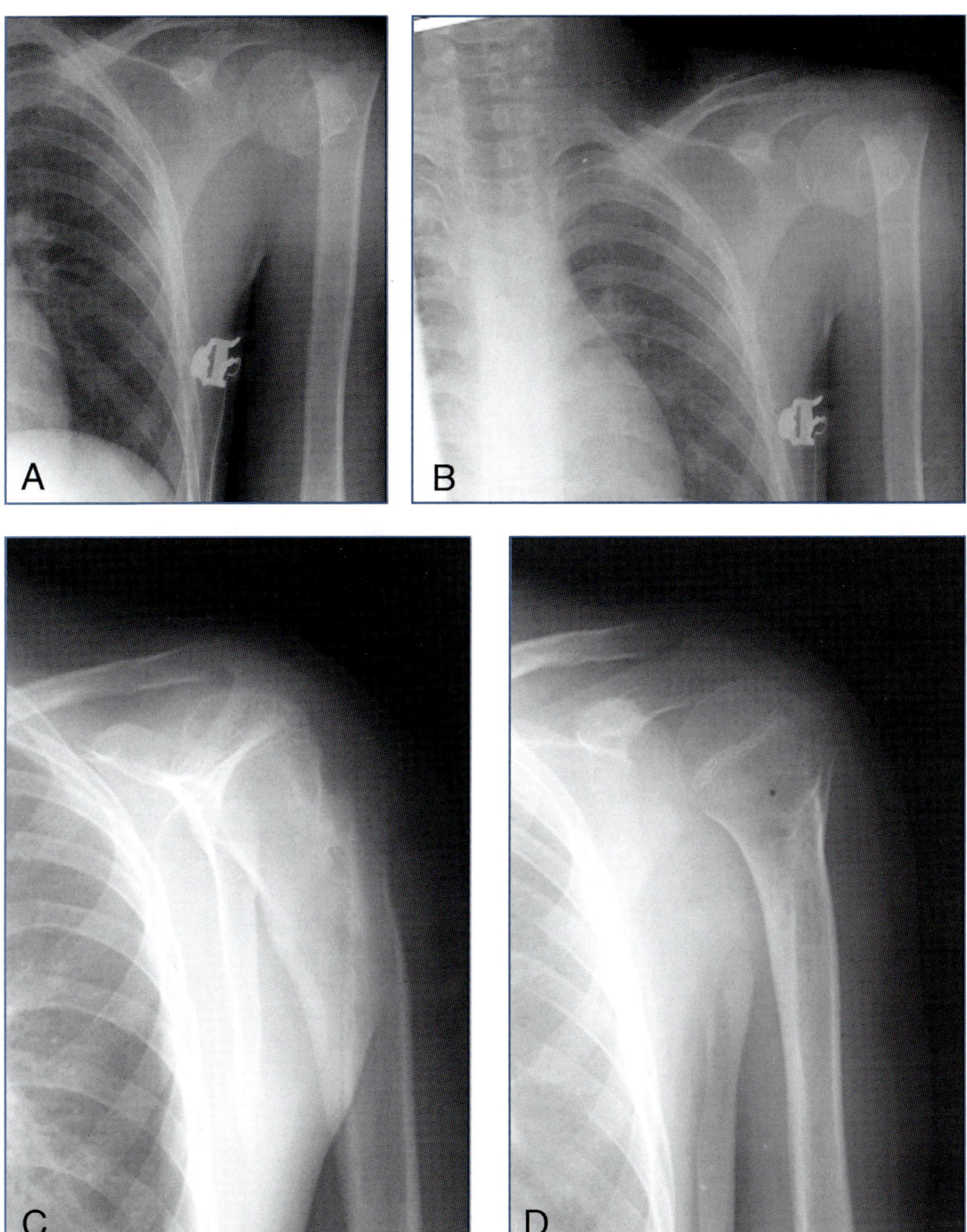

Figure 5 AP **(A)** and attempted lateral **(B)** radiographs show a completely displaced proximal humerus fracture in an 11-year-old boy. The fracture was immobilized with a sling and swathe for 4 weeks, followed by range-of-motion exercises. AP **(C)** and lateral **(D)** radiographs obtained 15 months after injury show excellent remodeling. The patient had no pain, lacked approximately 20° of shoulder elevation, and had normal shoulder internal and external rotation.

patient regained full range of motion in his shoulder within 3 months of the operation.

STRATEGIES TO MINIMIZE COMMON COMPLICATIONS

The vast majority of proximal humerus fractures in skeletally immature patients can and should be treated with immobilization alone (Figure 5). In some cases, closed reduction and immobilization is warranted. Although it is controversial, there are certain specific cases that warrant reduction and internal fixation of very displaced and angulated proximal humeral fractures in adolescents approaching skeletal maturity. In the case presented here, the fracture involved the dominant arm of a boy within 1 or 2 years of skeletal maturity. Attempts at closed reduction and immobilization failed to yield satisfactory alignment. An attempt at closed reduction and pinning failed because of the interposed biceps tendon and periosteum. An open reduction allowed removal of the interposed tissue. Percutaneous lateral pinning, with threaded pins and careful attention to pin placement, yielded an excellent result in this boy.

REFERENCES

1. Blount WP: *Fractures in Children.* Baltimore, MD, Williams & Wilkins, 1954.
2. Beringer DC, Weiner DS, Noble JS, Bell RH: Severely displaced proximal humeral epiphyseal fractures: A follow-up study. *J Pediatr Orthop* 1998;18:31-37.
3. Dobbs MB, Luhmann SL, Gordon JE, Strecker WB, Schoenecker PL: Severely displaced proximal humeral epiphyseal fractures. *J Pediatr Orthop* 2003;23:208-215.
4. Beaty JH: Fractures of the proximal humerus and shaft in children. *Instr Course Lect* 1992;41:369-372.
5. Visser JD, Rietberg M: Interposition of the tendon of the long head of biceps in fracture separation of the proximal humeral epiphysis. *Neth J Surg* 1980;32:12-15.

Index

Page numbers with *f* indicate figures; page numbers with *t* indicate tables.

G

H

I

J

K

L

M

N

O

P

R

S

T

U

V

X